MW00850902

# Insider's Guide
## *to*
# MAYO CLINIC

## Second Edition

### Expert Advice for Patients and Family from the Patient's Perspective

Dr. Ron Wolfson

Copyright © 2020 Ron Wolfson

All rights reserved.

No part of this publication may be reproduced or transmitted in any form or by any means graphic, electronic or mechanical, including photocopying, recording or by any information storage and retrieval system, without permission in writing from the publisher.

The Mayo Clinic and Rochester, Minnesota, is a dynamic place. Please note that all the information in this edition of "insider's Guide" is current as of September, 2020.

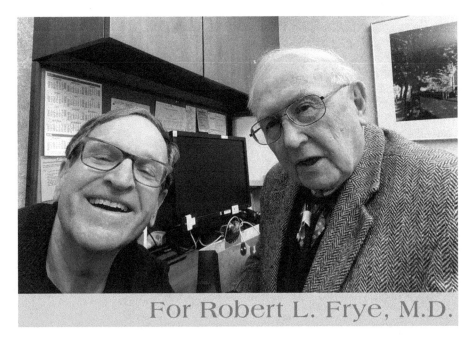

## For Robert L. Frye, M.D.

A physician scholar who epitomizes the values of Mayo Clinic and embodies the Hippocratic Oath: dedicated to "the art as well as the science of medicine, knowing that warmth, sympathy, and understanding outweigh the surgeon's knife or the chemist's drug; who is never ashamed to say 'I know not,' nor will fail to call in colleagues when the skills of another are needed for a patient's recovery; who does not treat a fever chart, a cancerous growth, but a sick human being, whose illness may affect the person's family and economic stability; who prevents disease whenever he can, for prevention is preferable to cure; who remains a member of society, with special obligations to all his fellow human beings, those sound of mind and body as well as the infirm."

Dr. Frye upholds his oath and has always acted to preserve the finest traditions of his calling. In return, may he always enjoy life and art, "respected while he lives and remembered with affection thereafter, and long experience the joy of healing those who seek his help."

# Contents

# Introduction

ONE DAY WHEN I WAS AT MAYO CLINIC WITH MY PARENTS, I said to their primary physician, Dr. Robert L. Frye: "You know, coming to Rochester and Mayo Clinic for the first time is like planning a trip to Disney World. You need to know where to stay, when to go, how to navigate the place, strategies for avoiding waiting in line, where to eat, and what to do if you have extra time." Dr. Frye said, "You know, Ron, that's a good point. How could we help people with that?" "Well," I responded, "the materials you prepare are excellent, the signage in the buildings is good, and everyone is friendly and helpful if people look lost. Yet for the first-timer at Mayo it is somewhat intimidating. The place is huge, and it takes some getting used to the Mayo model of care. What people could use is a guidebook written from the patient's point of view—like *Birnbaum's Guide to Disney World*." He looked me in the eye, smiled, and said, "Why don't you write it?"

Dr. Frye knew I was the author of eight books and an educator. I told him I was going on sabbatical from the university where I teach, and I would try my hand at it if I were given the blessing of the Clinic and offered cooperation during the research. After several months of vetting through the Mayo system, and with the encouragement of Dr. Frye, the senior administration agreed that such a guide would indeed be helpful to Mayo patients and their families.

The *Insider's Guide to Mayo Clinic* is the first book of its kind—a "travel guide," if you will, to one of the finest medical centers in the world. In fact, patients and their family members travel from all over the world, including Europe, Asia, Africa, Canada, North and South America, often with an unusual medical issue, hoping that they can find answers on the plains of southeastern Minnesota at the Rochester location—or at Mayo Clinic facilities in Phoenix/Scottsdale, Arizona, or Jacksonville, Florida (although this guide is specifically for Rochester).

The *Insider's Guide* was developed with the full cooperation of Mayo Clinic. They offered me complete access to physicians, administrators, and allied health staff. Every single interviewee was proud of the institution and supportive of the guide. They understood that the information gathered here will be helpful to the patients and families who choose to come to Mayo Clinic; and, as you will learn, at Mayo the needs of the patient come first.

This book would not have been possible without the enthusiastic support of Dr. Robert L. Frye, Professor of Medicine. He is the very embodiment of the Mayo model of care and compassion. Whenever our family has needed Dr. Frye he has responded immediately, including one memorable phone call from the Burgundy region of France. Our family has been forever enriched by his friendship and his skill. This book is dedicated to him with my deepest thanks.

I am grateful to all the wonderful people of Mayo who assisted me during my research and agreed to be interviewed as I sought to discover the "Insider Tips" about the Clinic experience: Dr. Eric Edell, Jill Buck, Matt Dacy, Amy Toberson, Becky Smith, Chris Askew, Gina Owens, Dr. James Hernandez, Dr. Patricia Simmons, Dr. Kaiser Lim, Judy Buckingham, Julie Lawson, Karen Fabian, Kent Seltman, Kim Keefe, Jenny Dusso, Michelle Leak, Rachel Bzoskie, Shelli Tradup, Barb Prigge, Randy Staver, and Jim Hodge.

I spoke to a number of Mayo patients on my visits to Rochester, including Don and Nancy Greenberg, Abe and Beverly Krasne, and others who did not wish to be identified by name. Their insights into the Mayo experience were invaluable.

The good people of Rochester are well represented by the terrific folks at the Rochester Convention and Visitors Bureau, including Brad Jones, Mary Gastner, and Darlene Aske, who generously provided their lodging and restaurant lists. John Wade at the Rochester Chamber of Commerce was supportive. Janelle Smith from Marquis Hospitality Group offered excellent insider tips.

I am grateful to Dr. Len Berry, Distinguished Marketing Professor at Texas A & M University, author of several important studies of the quality service model at Mayo, who validated the need for a guide of this kind.

A very special appreciation to Suzanne Leaf-Brock and Catherine Benson of Mayo Clinic's Division of Public Affairs, without whose encouragement and assistance I could never have written this guide. Catherine Stroebel provided excellent fact-checking to ensure accuracy of every detail of the Mayo experience.

The world-famous Mayo Clinic pioneered what I call "destination medicine". Organizing a visit to Mayo in Rochester, Minnesota, requires the same sort of preparation you would do for planning a trip to a destination resort. You need to answer these questions:

1. How do I get in?
2. When should I go?
3. Where can I stay?
4. Where do I eat?
5. What's there to do?
6. What's the weather like?

7. Will I have to wait around a lot?
8. What will it cost?

The *Insider's Guide to Mayo Clinic* provides answers to these questions and many more. All of the information in the guide is based on official policies and procedures of Mayo Clinic and has been fact-checked by the Clinic for accuracy at the time of publication. In addition, the Rochester Visitors and Convention Bureau has provided a complete listing of lodging alternatives for those traveling to Rochester to visit the Clinic. The "Insider Tips" in the Guide are solely based on my research and experience over more than twenty-five years of visits to Mayo, both as a family member accompanying a patient and as a patient myself.

Please check the *Insider's Guide to Mayo Clinic* website—www. clinicinsidersguide.com—for updated information, discussion boards, and other links to Mayo and Rochester information.

I vividly recall my first visits to Mayo and how overwhelmed I felt. My hope is that the *Insider's Guide* will help ease your way as you experience this remarkable place in a remarkable town—a place where you will encounter remarkable human beings who are passionate, caring, and dedicated to one thing: your health and well-being.

Welcome to Mayo Clinic!

# Chapter One "Take Me to Mayo"

MY FATHER-IN-LAW ABE IS ONE OF THE TOUGHEST GUYS YOU'LL EVER MEET. He lives in a Midwestern town in the home he has owned since 1956. His wife Hilde died sixteen years ago, so he lives alone. His only daughter, my wife Susie, lives in Los Angeles, a thousand miles away.

Abe has had his health issues. In 1991 he had open heart surgery in Los Angeles to replace a worn aortic heart valve and bypass five coronary arteries. He has chronic asthma and emphysema. Yet he is a vigorous man who lives by the slogan "Keep on moving." Every day since his retirement twenty years ago he drives to the local community center, where he works out for at least five hours each day. There he is known as "Mayor Abe," a legendary fixture at the health club. He literally runs circles around people half his age.

On April 12, 2005, Abe turned 95 years old. We celebrated his birthday in a car—on an emergency trip to Rochester, Minnesota . . . and Mayo Clinic.

Abe had fallen gravely ill. He had been admitted to a local hospital with a severe cough, shortness of breath, and extreme weakness. This incredibly physically fit man could not walk from one side of a room to the other. His doctor diagnosed congestive heart failure. When Abe asked what they could do, the doctor answered, "What do you want, Abe? You're ninety-five. Your

5

replacement heart valve was only good for at most ten years. It's been twelve years. There's nothing more to do."

"Take me to Mayo," Abe told us.

We called Dr. Robert Frye, an eminent cardiologist, who has been our family's Mayo doctor. Dr. Frye is the man who has kept my father Alan alive for more than twenty-six years after his major heart surgery at Mayo, a result that far exceeds the odds. Dr. Frye said what he always says when we call: "Bring him to Rochester."

And so, on a Sunday afternoon, we found ourselves driving east to Des Moines, and then heading north to Minnesota. Abe was slumped in the back seat, covered by a blanket, barely awake, extremely pale and getting weaker by the moment. We were in a race for his life—a race that took us to Mayo Clinic.

The drive took five hours or so of straight-line travel. A left turn at Des Moines, a right turn at Albert Lea, and a left turn just past Austin and the Spam Museum. You see nothing but cornfields and farms. And then suddenly, as you approach Rochester from the south on State Highway 63, you see it in the distance, rising from the hills like a medical Emerald City: the buildings of Mayo Clinic.

I glanced back at Dad, asleep against the back seat, and an over-whelming emotion engulfed every pore of my body. An emotional brew of hope, fear, excitement, and anxiety—conflicting feelings cascading over me like a waterfall. Above all I felt an eerie calm, knowing that we were taking Dad to Mayo to be seen by the finest physicians and medical professionals in the world. If there was any place that could give him another chance at life, it was here on the plains of southern Minnesota.

We drove up to Mayo Clinic's Saint Marys Hospital emergency department entrance, put Dad in a wheelchair selected from the dozens lined up for just this purpose, and approached the receptionist. It was Sunday night by now, and the waiting room was filled with at least thirty people in various states of illness and distress. The receptionist was a triage agent, responsible for assessing the severity of the presenting condition and recommending the appropriate attention. As soon as he learned that Dad was in heart failure, nurses were called and we were rushed into a treatment room.

Tests were conducted immediately, and the attending physician admitted Dad to the hospital. He was taken to the Cardiac Care Unit, where he was hooked up to high-tech heart monitoring equipment. We barely slept that night at the hotel across the street, hoping that the next day we would have some answer to our question: "Is there anything you can do to save his life?"

What we witnessed Monday morning in that hospital room was absolutely incredible. The cardiology team on call that day was led by Dr. Sabrina Phillips, a smartly dressed female cardiologist. She walked into Abe's room, introduced herself and her team of physicians with a warm greeting, and began to examine Dad. She listened to his heart and his lungs. She felt his feet and legs. And then she said, "Abe, let me see your fingers." Dad held out his hand for her to examine. The doctor took his hand in hers, looking carefully at his fingernails. In an instant she looked him straight in the eye and said, "Abe, you have an infection in your heart."

"What?" I exclaimed. "How do you know that?"

The doctor called me over to the bedside.

"See these red lines under his fingernails," she said as she held Dad's hand. "These are called splinter infractions. That's a sure indication that he has an infection somewhere in his heart. We'll have to take some blood samples and wait for the cultures to come back in a few days, but I'm certain that this is what is causing his heart failure. It could be an infection on his valve. Remember, it was replaced more than ten years ago, and that is the outside limit on porcine valves. In the meantime, Abe, we'll keep you comfortable by getting the swelling down, and then we'll see what our options might be."

No doctor had made a diagnosis like that. And the way she did it—by simply looking at his fingernails, like some sort of medical soothsayer! But this was no carnival arcade. This was Mayo Clinic. And we had faith that she would be right.

She was right. Abe had a severe infection of his aortic valve, the replaced valve. It was indeed giving out, having done its job for a good decade.

But what could be done, if anything?

Dr. Frye called Dr. Kenton Zehr, one of the Mayo cardiac thoracic surgeons, known for his willingness to assess patients on the basis of their condition, not their age. Dr. Zehr was compassionate—and blunt. "Your father needs a new valve or he will die. He is in excellent physical shape; I can see that. He wants to do the surgery; that's important. But I cannot do the surgery unless the infection clears up. I have consulted with Dr. Frye, and we have agreed on a course of treatment with powerful antibiotics. It will take at least eight weeks to clear up the infection— if it works. Then I want you to come back to the Clinic and we will re-evaluate."

A glimmer of hope.

We drove back home and admitted Dad to a rehabilitation center. The eight weeks seemed like a lifetime. The antibiotics were administered intravenously through a PIC line directly into his body. By June 1 Abe was ready to return to the Clinic to assess the infection.

Once again we drove the 350 miles to Rochester, this time with feelings of nervous optimism. If the infection had cleared up, there was a chance that the surgeon would consider doing the surgery. But would he risk it on a ninety-five-year-old man?

"There is good news," Dr. Frye said as we sat on the long couch in one of the examination rooms on the fifth floor of the Gonda Building. He looked at his computer screen displaying the results of an angiogram taken earlier that same day. "The infection is nearly gone. Dr. Zehr will meet with you at three p.m."

"I see you're back, Abe," Dr. Zehr greeted us. "I've looked at the test, and there is still a little residual material on the valve, but it is much better than before. The drugs did their job. Now the question is: Should we do the surgery? It's risky. I would estimate you have a fifteen percent chance of not making it off the table."

"Fifteen percent?" Dad said. "That's not bad. I'll take it. I can't live like this."

"No, you can't, "Dr. Zehr agreed. "Your prognosis is not good unless we can put a new valve in there. Are you certain you want to go ahead with this?"

"Absolutely sure," Dad said.

"Okay then. Let me look at my schedule," Dr. Zehr said, pulling out a little black book. "I can do it in three weeks—June 24."

"I'll be here." Dad smiled and shook the good doctor's hand. "There's just one thing. I bought a new car for my ninety-fifth birthday . . . and I insisted on a ten-year warranty. Can you give me the same deal on the heart valve?"

Dr. Zehr howled with laughter. "You bet we will, Abe!"

Once again we drove back home to await the appointed time. And once again, we drove back to Rochester, this time filled with anticipation.

The surgery was a complete success. Dad made a remarkable recovery–so much so that it seemed as if all the Mayo doctors and nurses came to see this ninety-five-year-old who was up out of bed within forty-eight hours after the operation and was walking around the floor in three days! There are no words to describe how grateful we were to Dr. Zehr, Dr. Frye, and their team.

We returned home with a new man who had a new heart and a new lease on life.

The recovery from the surgery proceeded well—until one day Abe developed a deep cough again and severe swelling of the limbs, sure indications that he was back in congestive heart failure. We rushed him to a local hospital, where the doctors diagnosed what they thought was a leak in the heart. Abe was in critical condition. He was put on a heart pump. The doctors held out little hope.

This was a complete surprise—and we called Dr. Zehr for a second opinion. After all, he had done the surgery on the heart just three weeks earlier.

"Bring him here. I'll send an air ambulance."

In three hours, the Mayo MedAir team arrived to take Dad back to Rochester, this time by medical jet. Susie and I drove in the car, yet another five-hour journey of fear and hope.

Once back at Saint Marys Hospital, Dr. Zehr and Dr. Frye ordered a battery of tests to determine what was happening. There was no leak; Abe's condition was severe congestive heart failure, most likely brought on by an imbalance of fluid intake and diuretics. There was no need for additional surgery.

In short order Dad recovered well. As of this writing, a year later, he is back full-time at the health club, driving his ten-year-warranty car, tending to the sixty tomato plants in his garden, and enjoying the new lease on life granted by Mayo Clinic.

# The Mayo Model of Care

Mayo Clinic is routinely rated as one of the top medical centers in the world. Although it is located in a relatively remote area of the United States, more than one million unique patient visits are made at the original Clinic facility in Rochester, Minnesota, each year. Most of these patients come to Rochester with at least one family member, leading to the amazing fact that this small city of 110,000 plays host to millions of visitors a year! That puts Rochester in the top ten tourist sites in America!

Everything in Rochester is organized brilliantly to facilitate patients and their families' needs. From the wide variety of accommodations ranging from budget to luxurious to the convenience of shuttle vans from virtually every hotel to the Clinic and hospitals to the special diet menus offered in many restaurants, nothing has been left to chance.

Yet during my many interviews of patients and family members I heard one refrain over and over again that explains why people love Mayo Clinic: the personal care they feel from everyone they meet.

11

In the Clinic you see this every day, nearly every minute. Standing at the geographic hub of the sprawling downtown complex—the Subway level of the spectacular new Gonda Building—it is not unusual to witness patients and accompanying family members with a computerized appointment schedule printout in hand, looking absolutely lost, befuddled about which way to turn to go to Hilton Building Desk C or where to find Station S or which elevator to take to Mayo 5 East.

Yet, within seconds a volunteer, an escort, or even a doctor—anyone who wears the ubiquitous black name tag on his or her breast pocket—will approach someone with that "look of lost" on their face and offer assistance. This is no accident; every staff member is trained to look for the "look" and to respond immediately, creating an "ambience of care" that permeates the entire institution.

This ambience of care is at the core of Mayo Clinic Mission Statement and Core Values, first articulated by Dr. William J. Mayo:

"THE BEST INTERESTS OF THE PATIENT ARE THE ONLY INTERESTS TO BE CONSIDERED . . ."

For all the attention to cutting-edge medical research and practice, the folks at Mayo never lose sight of the *reason* they are there: to serve the patient, to welcome the family, and to offer the highest quality experience of healing. In short, at Mayo Clinic *"the needs of the patient come first."*

I asked the father of a first-time patient to describe the Mayo experience:

> I sent an email to Mayo through their online website (www.mayoclinic.org). I was looking for doctors on the front lines and in the trenches. I liked the team approach. I wanted a place where doctors weren't

afraid to say "I don't know, but I'll ask my colleague." I wanted to learn more about my son's disease. Our doctor at home had seen his condition only once before; here at Mayo, they've seen it thirty-five times in eighty years, so it's pretty rare.

Mayo is a humanly efficient place. I couldn't believe it when every single time I called to arrange our visit, a real human being answered. Where in the world today can you call and not push numbers to get recordings of information? Everything they told us would be here is here. I have confidence in this place.

Yes, it's enormous. Yes, it can be a little intimidating your first day here. But the signs are good, and the people are nice. I never felt stupid asking a question; everyone treated every question with respect.

This carried over into the tests themselves. You're nervous, you know, when doing a CAT scan. But the instructions were given to my son simply, directly— he knew when he could breathe, when he could swallow, when he had to be still, and when he could move.

I'm very pleased we chose Mayo. This is the Mecca of medicine.

Mayo's style of medicine is based on the three-fold mission of the Clinic represented by the three shields in the Mayo logo—clinical practice, research, and education—and rooted in these unusual factors:

1. Everyone is on salary.

At Mayo Clinic no one has any financial motivation to suggest anything other than procedures and medications that will benefit the patient. There is no monetary gain to any individual for recommending a surgery or *not* recommending a surgery. You will receive the best advice from top health professionals who have no monetary incentive whatsoever. In today's health care climate, this is highly unusual.

2. You will never be rushed.

At Mayo Clinic you will never be hurried out of a consultation with a doctor or other health professional. They will give you whatever time you need to fully understand your diagnosis and your instructions for treatment. You will have time to get answers to all of your questions. In fact, Mayo folks are so thorough, they will read the look on your face to make sure you understand what's being said–and if you don't understand, they will elaborate until you do. How unusual is that?

3. Your case will *not* be unusual.

With more than one million outpatient visits each year in the Clinic, the Mayo doctors have seen just about every possible medical condition and complication known to humankind. In the typical medical center, even in mid-size or large communities, rare diseases and conditions are rarely seen. At Mayo Clinic every department will see dozens of cases involving rare diseases. This happens because many physicians from all over the world refer their patients with rare conditions to Mayo Clinic for evaluation and treatment.

4. The doctors collaborate with each other.

The Mayo brothers invented the concept of group medicine. They insisted that every physician, specialist, resident, intern, and nurse contribute to the deliberation that results in diagnosis and recommended treatment. If a physician is puzzled, the culture encourages her/him to admit "I don't know" and to consult colleagues who do. Moreover, every single professional who sees you at the Clinic records his or her observations in an electronic chart, a database that is instantly available via a computer intranet to those responsible for your care at Mayo. Their commitment is to get to the bottom of what's happening with you. Alan Wolfson says: "At Mayo Clinic, the M.D. after the doctor's name stands for 'Medical Detective.'"

5. You can accomplish in a week at Mayo what would take months to do almost anywhere else.

When you come to Mayo Clinic, everything necessary for a complete diagnosis is available in one location. If your primary physician needs you to have a CAT scan, you will have one scheduled within days, not weeks or months. If you need to see a specialist, one will be called in on your case immediately; you will not need to wait weeks or months. When you give a blood sample, you do not wait hours or days for the results; they are ready almost instantaneously. As Don Greenberg, a Mayo patient, told me, "Instead of running around my home town for weeks, I had 100% of the tests done to diagnose my condition in two days at Mayo. I arrived on Sunday night, had tests on Monday and Tuesday, by Wednesday there was a diagnosis, and on Friday of the same week I had surgery. Where else in the world can you get all that done in such a short amount of time?"

6. Staff members are highly skilled at what they do.

Have you ever had a technician try to draw a blood sample from your arm who couldn't find a vein? Were you poked two or three times? I was traumatized as a child when a novice nurse stuck my chubby little arms endlessly until she penetrated a vein. This is nearly unheard of at Mayo Clinic. A crew drawn from six hundred expert phlebotomists do nothing all day but draw blood from patients. The same can be said of the technicians who work in radiology, the physician assistants who dispense chemotherapy, and the staff who operate the dialysis machines—not to mention the highly skilled nurses who assist surgeons in the operating room who remain largely unseen by patients and their families. These people know their business.

Incredibly, there are *fourteen* allied-health professionals for every one of the 1,734 physicians and scientists at Mayo Clinic. Each person is considered a valuable asset and contributes immeasurably to the culture of caring that defines the place. Examples abound of strong institutional loyalty and long years of service; there is a very low turnover rate. It is not unusual to find staff who have worked at the Clinic for 20, 30 or more years.

7. Practice is informed by research.

A significant portion of the annual $5 billion operating budget of Mayo Clinic is devoted to medical research. Clinical trials of the latest medicines and therapies are routinely performed here. Breakthroughs are commonplace, and the latest medical knowledge is immediately applied to patient care. Dr. Eric Edell says, "We're always working on an answer we don't yet have. We're always asking what we can do tomorrow. There is always the hope for advances in medicine. That is why Mayo is so committed to research."

8. The doctors, nurses, and researchers are teachers.

Mayo is a teaching place. Many of the clinical physicians are also scholar-practitioners, pursuing their areas of interest and pushing forward the boundaries of medical knowledge. If you are admitted to one of the hospitals, you will likely be seen by a team of doctors, including residents and/or medical students who are led by a senior Mayo consultant physician. There are five education programs: Mayo Medical School (for beginning physicians), Mayo Graduate School of Medicine (for residents learning a specialty), Mayo Graduate School (for researchers), Mayo School of Health Related Sciences (for allied health providers such as nurses and therapists), and Mayo School of Continuing Medical Education (for those health professionals seeking professional development education opportunities).

9. Midwestern people are genuinely nice.

There is truth to the reputation that the people of Mayo Clinic are "Minnesota nice." Having been born and raised in a great Midwestern town, and having lived in Southern California for thirty-two years, I know from where I speak. There is a no-nonsense, straight-shooting, values-driven culture among the people who live and work in Rochester that shapes the entire experience of being there. These folks are hard-working and efficient, yet compassionate and caring. They confront the challenges, successes, and failures of medicine daily with a deep-seated passion for healing. They are not superhuman; they are real.

10. You can establish a lifelong relationship with this place for your complex medical problems

Patients come to Mayo Clinic for a one-time evaluation or treatment. My family, however, is an example of making Mayo Clinic their go-to center for serious illness. My grandmother Ida Paperny had the first vaginal hysterectomy performed at Mayo—and paid for the surgery by sending a $1 bill in an envelope to "Dr. Mayo, Rochester, Minnesota" every Friday for years. My grandfather Louis had a check-up at Mayo every year. My mother was treated there as an adolescent, and my father's heart surgery twenty-six years ago—and the subsequent care offered by Mayo—has enabled him to reach the age of eighty-five. This is not true just for those who live within driving distance of Rochester; there are patients who literally travel the world to seek the very special care offered at Mayo whenever a complex medical need arises. They must know something.

The Mayo model of care is the bedrock foundation of the institution, a model of care that ensures that when you come to Mayo you will receive outstanding medical treatment within a culture of caring that is second to none in the world.

## The Mayo Family

How one family doctor and his sons created the foundation for a world-class medical center on the plains of Minnesota is truly one of the most remarkable stories in American history. Dr. William Worrall Mayo came from England to the United States in 1846 and graduated from Indiana Medical College in 1850. He and his wife Louise Wright Mayo settled in Minnesota in 1854.

Working as a Civil War examining surgeon, he moved his family to Rochester in 1863. Their two sons, Dr. William James Mayo and Dr. Charles Horace Mayo, joined the practice in 1883 and 1888. Together the doctors Mayo pioneered a system of health care that revolutionized medicine.

The doctors Mayo had partners. After a devastating tornado destroyed much of Rochester in 1883, Mother Alfred Moes and Sister Mary Joseph Dempsey, leaders of the Sisters of St. Francis, were asked to care for the injured. Mother Alfred Moes proposed to build and staff a hospital if Dr. Mayo and his sons would provide the medical care. Saint Marys Hospital opened in 1889. Physicians from neighboring communities were invited to join them, laying the groundwork for a group practice. One of these partners, Dr. Henry Plummer, was an organizational genius, designing and creating buildings and systems that facilitated critical communication among the doctors in the growing integrated practice. Combining medical practice and education, the doctors Mayo and their associates quickly gained a nationwide reputation as a place of inquiry, research, and excellence in care for patients. The teamwork, exchange of ideas, and reflective practice led to the name "Mayo Clinic".

The expanding practice required new facilities. In 1914, the first building designed for the integrated practice of medicine was built. In 1928, the efficient architectural masterpiece known as the Plummer Building was completed, and it housed much of the Clinic's work until 1955. The Mayo Building opened then, and it was expanded between 1966 and 1970. Additional buildings were constructed for the Clinic, along with Rochester Methodist Hospital (1954). The Gonda Building was dedicated in 2001.

The Mayo commitment to medical education began with the establishment of the Mayo Graduate School of Medicine in 1915, and since then more than 17,000 doctors have served as graduate residents in the Clinic, learning their specialties. Physicians in training, called "fellows," joined the Mayo partners in learning medical specialties. In 1972, the Mayo Medical School opened for the undergraduate preparation of physicians.

Medical research has been a hallmark of Mayo. In addition to pioneering techniques in patient treatment and surgery, Mayo staff have invented medical equipment and formulated important pharmaceuticals, and in 1950 Drs. Kendall and Hench shared the Nobel Prize for their development of cortisone.

The most amazing achievement of all, however, may have come when the Mayo Brothers, Dr. Will and Dr. Charlie, bequeathed their practice to the future, creating a nonprofit foundation to sustain the legacy of their family. In 1939, on the eve of World War II, Dr. Will, Dr. Charlie, and Sister Mary Joseph Dempsey died, all in the same year. Yet the foundation of Mayo Clinic had been well laid. Their successors have built a world-renowned group medical practice with three locations, in Rochester, Jacksonville and Phoenix/Scottsdale, that attracts patients from all parts of the globe. You are about to join the more than seven million people who have come to this place seeking diagnosis, treatment, and healing.

For more on the history of Mayo Clinic, visit the various historical displays and museums on campus and in the hospitals, click on www.mayoclinic.org/tradition-heritage/, and consider reading the classic book by Helen Clapesattle, *The Doctors Mayo*.

# Chapter Two What Is Mayo Clinic?

MAYO CLINIC IS THE COMMON NAME USED TO REFER TO THE MEDICAL COMMUNITY of health professionals and researchers in Rochester, Minnesota, and two branches of the Clinic in Jacksonville, Florida, and Phoenix/Scottsdale, Arizona.

The two main points of connection for patients in Rochester are:

**Mayo Clinic**—an outpatient "clinic" where individuals see Mayo physicians and receive diagnostic tests and medical treatment;

**Saint Marys Campus** (often referred to as **"Saint Marys Hospital**), **Mayo Eugenio Litta Children's Hospital** (located within Saint Marys) and **Methodist Campus** (often referred to as **"Rochester Methodist Hospital"**)—the three hospitals that are owned and operated by Mayo to serve those individuals who need "inpatient" medical treatment.

Most patients are seen as "outpatients," meaning they do not stay at the hospital. The "clinic" is not one big room; there are more than eighty buildings in the "Mayo Clinic"! You receive a schedule of appointments, tests, and treatments that are done at the main Mayo Clinic buildings downtown; ninety percent of these appointments are seen in the two largest outpatient Clinic buildings—the Mayo Building and the Gonda Building. At the end of your day at the Clinic, you return to your home or lodging.

## When Do You Need Mayo Clinic?

Mayo Clinic is an excellent choice when a person has been diagnosed with a serious medical condition by a local physician and he or she seeks to confirm the diagnosis and/or get a second opinion. If your doctor suspects a rare disease, Mayo Clinic has most likely seen a number of cases of virtually every medical anomaly known to humankind. The Clinic has limited capacity for patients requesting a general physical examination or for treatment of routine illnesses. In fact, Mayo recommends that your routine, acute and primary care needs be handled by your regular physician at home whenever possible because long-distance care for such matters is not in your best interest. In addition, there is more demand for Mayo appointments than capacity, but the Clinic does its best to see all who need its services. If the Rochester campus cannot accommodate you, try the excellent—and rapidly expanding—Mayo Clinic facilities and staff in Phoenix/Scottsdale, Arizona, and Jacksonville, Florida.

In many cases Mayo is seen as the last stop on a medical journey. However, in the case of a cancer diagnosis, the Clinic would rather see you as soon as possible—before treatment begins elsewhere—in order to prescribe the best course of therapy.

### Insider Tip

Chris Askew, coordinator of volunteer services, recognizes that many patients who come to Mayo Clinic have been told they have a major threat to their health and are coming for a second opinion, looking for answers and a solution to the problem. They are seeking hope, coming with the expectation: "If they can't fix it at Mayo, they can't fix it anywhere."

Mayo does operate a regional health network of clinics serving the population of southeastern Minnesota called Mayo Health System.

## Isn't It Too Expensive to Go to Mayo?

The answer is "no." Medical care at Mayo Clinic is no more costly than at any other major medical center in the United States. In fact, in some cases the costs are lower than those of medical care in large urban clinics and hospitals.

There is, of course, extra cost whenever you travel to a "destination medicine" center. The expenses for gas, airplane tickets, rental cars, hotels, and food can add up. But the cost is outweighed by the relative speed of getting all of your diagnostic tests and treatments done in a concentrated period of time in one of the top medical centers in the world.

## Mayo Clinic, Rochester, Minnesota

Mayo Clinic and the Mayo Clinic Hospitals form an integrated medical center dedicated to providing comprehensive diagnosis and treatment in virtually every medical and surgical specialty.

# Getting In

There are two unfortunate misconceptions about "getting in" to Mayo Clinic: 1) It is difficult to get an appointment at Mayo Clinic, and 2) You need a doctor's referral to get in. **Fully 60% of patients "self-refer" to Mayo, while 40% are referred by local physicians.** And while it may take some time to schedule an appointment with a particular department (for example, getting an orthopedics or sleep clinic appointment may take six months) or a specific doctor, if you really want to "get in" to Mayo, there are several ways to do so:

## 1. Physician's Referral

Perhaps the best way to enter the Clinic is through your local physician's referral. Doctors routinely advise their patients to seek evaluations and/or second opinions. Ideally, your physician will know of a specific doctor or department to call. The Mayo doctors want to respond to requests from their colleagues. Physicians are encouraged to make appointments for their patients by calling Mayo Clinic Referring Physicians Service and can find the info they need to make a referral by visiting http://www.mayoclinic.org/medicalprofs-rst. Your physician will need to provide the prospective patient's name, address, phone number, date of birth, Mayo Clinic registration number (if a previous patient), type and name of insurance, nature of medical problem or diagnosis, physician's UPIN, services you expect from Mayo, and a list of testing that has been done. Your physician can speak with a Mayo doctor twenty-four hours a day, seven days a week, by calling

1-800-533-1564. (This service is available only to physicians; patients seeking appointments, see below.)

## Insider Tip

The appointment calendars for most departments open ninety days in advance, so plan accordingly to call twelve weeks before you hope to come to the Clinic. Depending on medical need, some appointments may be triaged to an earlier date if an appointment slot is available.

You will be invited to bring along your medical records from your local physician, although it may be necessary for some tests to be repeated when you are at the Clinic in order for the Mayo doctors to have a "baseline" in accordance with their laboratory standards.

## Insider Tip

*"But I don't want my local doctor upset that I'm going to Mayo. I'm afraid I'll hurt his/her feelings."* Do local doctors feel jealous if you decide to go to Mayo? Perhaps, but it's your life, and you are entitled to a second opinion. You may find that the Mayo diagnosis and treatment plan is exactly the same as that suggested by the local physician. Then you gain tremendous peace of mind by having the situation confirmed by Mayo and a feeling of confidence that the local doctor is following a plan that has been validated by another source.

## 2. Making an Appointment Yourself

You can make an appointment at the Clinic on your own. Call the general number for Mayo, 507-284-2111, and ask for the Appointment Information Desk. You will speak with Jill Buck's well-trained staff, who will ask you questions about they type of care you are seeking—the main reason you want to come to Mayo—as well as insurance information and your demographic information. It's important that you share your medical concerns at the time of this conversation. The staff person will check for availability for your most pressing issues and tell you on the spot when you can get in, if you will be placed on a waitlist, or if they do not have an appointment to offer you. You will also be offered help in determining how to get to Rochester, Minnesota, types of lodging available, and other important logistical information.

International and non-English-speaking patients can call a dedicated appointment phone line at 507-284-8884, fax 507-538-3891, or access the website, www.mayoclinic.org/international.

### Insider Tip

There is no one good time to call for appointment. Calendars in different specialties open at different times during the year.

This main call center receives more than 312,000 phone calls per year. That's 6,000 phone calls a week, so it's a good idea to plan when you will call.

The Appointment Information Desk is open from 7:00 a.m. to 7:00 p.m. Monday through Thursday and from 7:00 a.m. to 6:00 p.m. on Friday.

Alternatively, you can request an appointment online at www.mayoclinic.org.

## Insider Tip

Call volume is heaviest between 9:00 a.m. and 2:30 p.m. and between 4:00 p.m. and 5:00 p.m. Central time. The best time to call is early morning between 7:00 a.m. and 9:00 a.m. or between 2:30 p.m. and 4:00 p.m.

## Insider Tip

If you know the name of a particular physician, you can call the main Mayo number and request to speak to her/his appointment secretary. Or you may call the Mayo operator and ask for the offices in each subspecialty. You can then ask for an appointment, and if there are openings, you may receive one. However, for first-timers it is best to call the Appointment Information Desk, since they have the "big picture" of what appointments are available in every department and for every physician.

## Insider Tip

You can find a list of all the Mayo physicians in Rochester by going online to **www.mayoclinic.org**, then clicking on the link for Mayo Clinic, Rochester, MN. Then, click on "Find a medical department or center." Once you click on the department you want, click on "Doctors" to see a list of all the physicians.

## 3. Executive Health Program

Mayo offers a "fast-track" comprehensive medical evaluation program for busy executives that provides a comprehensive medical evaluation within two days. Participants meet with an internal medicine specialist on the first day of the visit who conducts an initial examination, schedules consultations and tests, and reviews all results and recommended treatment and follow-up. Age and gender appropriate preventative services are provided. This may include screening for early detection of cancer and heart disease through laboratory tests, mammogram, colon imaging, and cardiovascular health consult with treadmill stress test. These physicians review your medications, assess your approach to stress management, alcohol, tobacco, personal safety, and risk of disease from your family history. Other medical concerns may also be addressed during this visit. Immunizations are updated. A detailed report including final recommendations and laboratory tests is issued to you, not the company. Most patients arrive on the day before their appointments, since medical tests begin at 7:00 a.m. An Executive Health Program coordinator is available to answer questions. Both men and women are welcome; spouses of executives who may wish to enter the Clinic are usually accommodated. There is a $1,100 administrative fee for admission to the program; average costs range from $5,000 - $12,000. For more information or reservations, call 507-284-2288 or email ExecutiveHealth@mayo.edu.

**Insider Tip**

If time is of the essence, this is the quickest way to complete an evaluation at Mayo Clinic. All three Mayo Clinic sites—Rochester, Jacksonville and Phoenix/ Scottsdale—offer the program. Appointments can be scheduled up to one year in advance, and scheduling well ahead of when you wish to visit is encouraged.

**Insider Tip**

Like most not-for-profit organizations, Mayo Clinic depends on the generosity of donors to support its mission. For information contact Department of Development, 507-284-8540, 800-297-1185, or email development@mayo.edu.

4. Women's Heart Clinic

Mayo offers a comprehensive Women's Heart Clinic offering full access to cardiovascular diagnoses and treatment options. Patients complete a questionnaire prior to admission to identify risk factors for diseases common to women. During the initial cardiac exam, Women's Heart Clinic cardiologists review your medical history and order diagnostic tests. Physicians may refer you, or you may request an appointment by calling 507-538-6857.

5. Unscheduled Appointment

Although it is not a good idea, some patients do show up at the Mayo Clinic without a scheduled appointment. Go directly to the Admissions and Business Services Desk in the lobby of the Gonda Building. From there you will be directed to the Unscheduled Appointment Area, where a staff member will meet you and arrange for a nurse to assess your medical condition (this process is called "triage"). If you are not in need of emergency care, you will likely need to wait several days for your first scheduled appointment. However, this depends on how busy the Clinic is at the time, the number of cancellations, and the urgency of your medical needs. If you want some idea of your chances, call the main Clinic number at 507-284-2111, and they can identify the anticipated wait time.

You may be given a pager or advised of a time to return to check on when you can be seen. As soon as an appointment becomes available, you will be referred to a medical area to begin your evaluation. You may see a physician or a mid-level provider (a nurse practitioner or physician's assistant who is supervised by a physician). You will always be given the name and phone number of a Patient Relations representative who can answer your questions as you wait for entry into the Clinic.

### Insider Tip

You'll have a better chance of "getting in" without a previously scheduled appointment during the winter months November—March.

## 6. Emergency

If you have a medical emergency, go immediately to the Emergency Department at Saint Marys Hospital. Once there, you will have your medical condition assed by a triage nurse. If you are in a life-threatening situation, you will be treated immediately. You may or may not be admitted to the hospital. If you are not in immediate danger, you will likely wait a period of time to be seen by a doctor.

## Insider Tip

If you are admitted to one of the hospitals, you are effectively "in" Mayo Clinic. You will be seen by Mayo physicians while you are in the hospital, and you will be scheduled for follow-up appointments as an outpatient, if necessary.

# When to Go

### 1. Hours

The main patient care buildings of Mayo Clinic are generally open from 6:30 a.m. to 6:30 p.m. Monday through Friday. The Clinic is closed on major holidays. The hospitals, of course, operate twenty-four hours per day, every day of the year.

### 2. The Subway/Skyway System

Mayo Clinic buildings are clustered in downtown Rochester in an eight-block area. Most of the buildings are connected by an underground tunnel system called the "Subway." No, there are no trains in this Subway! "Sub" means it's underground, and "way" means there are halls to get from one building to another. Think of it as a series of corridors linking the basement levels of the buildings.

In addition to the Subway, there is a "Skyway" system linking the Mayo buildings with surrounding buildings in downtown Rochester. These are pedestrian bridges that connect the buildings, providing climate-controlled passage over the streets below.

Speaking of climate, the main reason for the Subway/Skyway system is for patients and staff to get to their appointments without hazarding the often extreme temperatures and weather in Rochester. Neither cold, nor heat, nor rain, nor wind, nor snow will prevent you from your appointed tests and consultations!

### Insider Tip

Once in the Subway/Skyway system, it is easy to get turned around, walk in circles or even get lost. Use a map that indicates the corridors in the Subway/ Skyway and look for directional signs at key intersections. There are also maps of the system at various locations throughout the corridors.

### Insider Tip

You don't need to wear huge coats at the Clinic, even in the winter. You can get to every place in the heated Subway/Skyway if you stay downtown. Of course, you'll need a coat to go outside in the winter; there are coat rooms available to check it.

The good folks of Rochester who own businesses catering to Mayo patients are enthusiastic supporters of the Subway/Skyway system. It enables visitors to reach hotels,

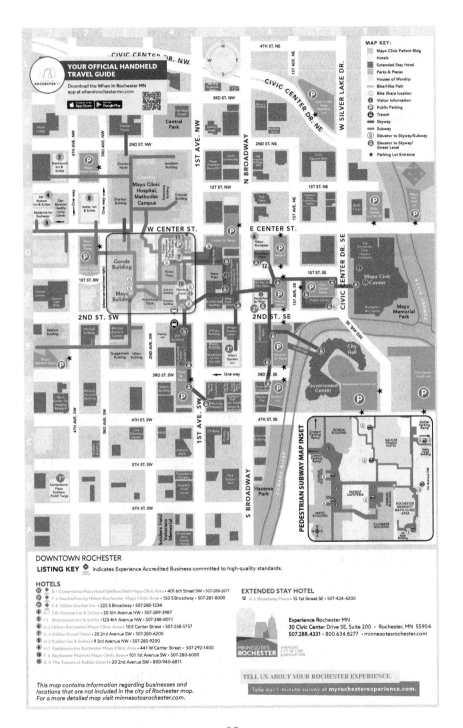

## DOWNTOWN ROCHESTER

**LISTING KEY** ✦ Indicates Experience Accredited Business committed to high-quality standards.

### HOTELS

1. B-1 Centerstone Plaza Hotel Soldiers Field-Mayo Clinic Area • 401 6th Street SW • 507-288-2677
2. F-6 DoubleTree by Hilton Rochester -Mayo Clinic Area • 150 S Broadway • 507-281-8000
3. F-5 Hilton Garden Inn • 225 S Broadway • 507-285-1234
4. H-1 5th Avenue Inn & Suites • 20 5th Avenue NW • 507-289-3987
5. J-1 Brentwood Inn & Suites •123 4th Avenue NW • 507-288-8011
6. G-5 Hilton Rochester/Mayo Clinic Area • 10 E Center Street • 507-258-5757
7. G-4 Kahler Grand Hotel • 20 2nd Avenue SW • 507-280-6200
8. H-2 Kahler Inn & Suites • 9 3rd Avenue NW • 507-285-9200
9. H-1 Residence Inn Rochester Mayo Clinic Area • 441 W Center Street • 507-292-1400
10. F-6 Rochester Marriott Mayo Clinic Area • 101 1st Avenue SW • 507-280-6000
11. G-4 The Towers at Kahler Grand • 20 2nd Avenue SW • 800-940-6811

### EXTENDED STAY HOTEL

12. G-6 Broadway Plaza • 15 1st Street SE • 507-424-4200

**Experience Rochester MN**
30 Civic Center Drive SE, Suite 200 • Rochester, MN 55904
507.288.4331 • 800.634.8277 • minnesotasrochester.com

MINNESOTA'S **ROCHESTER** AMERICA'S CITY OF CARE & INNOVATION

*This map contains information regarding businesses and locations that are not included in the city of Rochester map. For a more detailed map visit minnesotasrochester.com.*

**TELL US ABOUT YOUR ROCHESTER EXPERIENCE**

Take our 1-minute survey at **myrochesterexperience.com.**

restaurants, banks, and shops in comfort any time of the year. The Subway/Skyway system is indicated on the map by green corridors and dotted lines between buildings. In most patient care buildings the Subway Level is reached by elevator by pushing the "S" button.

## 3. Seasons/Weather

Rochester is located on the plains of southeastern Minnesota, a place that is blessed with the four seasons. Average temperatures/precipitation by month are:

|  | JAN | FEB | MAR | APR | MAY | JUNE | JULY | AUG | SEPT | OCT | NOV | DEC |
|---|---|---|---|---|---|---|---|---|---|---|---|---|
| High | 20 | 26 | 39 | 55 | 68 | 77 | 80 | 78 | 69 | 57 | 39 | 24 |
| Low | 4 | 11 | 23 | 35 | 46 | 56 | 60 | 58 | 49 | 37 | 24 | 10 |
| Precip. | .94 | .75 | 1.88 | 3.01 | 3.53 | 4.0 | 4.61 | 4.33 | 3.12 | 2.20 | 2.01 | 1.02 |

The coldest month is January; the warmest and wettest month is July. The all-time high temperature was 108 degrees in 1956; the coldest temperature on record: -42 degrees in 1887. The cold months of November through March require extensive use of the Subway/Skyway system. If you decide to stay at lodging that is not connected to the Clinic buildings, you will need to transition from your hotel to the shuttle bus in very cold weather.

## 4. Tips on Timing

The most important thing to know when planning a visit to Mayo is that virtually everything except for the hospitals shuts down over the weekend. The Clinic offices are closed, as are many of the businesses in the Subway corridors that cater to Mayo patients and family members.

This means that if you are not finished with your schedule of appointments on Friday, you will likely be staying in Rochester over the weekend. While there is plenty to do in

Rochester and the surrounding area (see below), you will not be able to see doctors or take tests (unless you are admitted to the hospital). Beginning on Thursday, some local patients head home for the weekend. Because they live within driving distance, they can come back for appointments the following week. Often, though not always, this can open up appointment slots for those who stand by. Curiously, a similar dynamic often results in appointment slots opening up on Mondays.

### Insider Tip

The day (or Friday) before a major holiday–New Year's Eve, Easter, Memorial Day, Independence Day, Labor Day, Thanksgiving, Christmas—appointment traffic is light in the Clinic.

### Insider Tip

In years past, the Clinic was not as busy during the winter months, November through March. Clinic administrators have noted that usage patterns have evened out somewhat as patients realize that they can get around the Clinic without ever having to step outside, especially if you stay in a downtown hotel connected to the Clinic by the Subway/Skyway system. The summer months are the busiest time of the year at Mayo.

## 5. How Long Will My Visit Be?

There is no telling in advance how long your visit at Mayo Clinic will be. It depends on the number of consultations, the tests ordered by the physicians, and the time it takes to get test results. A medical evaluation can usually be offered within three to six working days. Yet savvy insiders will tell you to plan on a longer stay—just in case. There is a kind of "snowball effect" as one test result may lead to the need for a further test. As one veteran says, "Come prepared to stay as long as it takes to get your answer." You are better off making arrangements to take care of the kids, the pets, and work for at least a week to be safe; the alternative will cause you to scramble at a time when you may be under stress in any case.

## 6. Canceling an Appointment

If for some reason you need to cancel an appointment at the Clinic, you should call the phone number on your appointment confirmation letter or the Appointment Information Desk, 507-284-2111.

### Insider Tip

If you are calling any phone number within Mayo from a Clinic phone, you need only dial the last five digits of the number.

## Preparing to Go

### 1. Your Medical Records

It is a good idea to bring along or send ahead medical records, lab results and copies of X rays from your local physician. If these records are mailed, be sure to put your

Mayo physician's name or at minimum the specialty area on the envelope; if they get sent to "Mayo Clinic" they may not end up where they need to be in a timely manner. These records are reviewed by the Mayo doctors as they look at your medical history.

### Insider Tip

Dr. James Hernandez, chair of Mayo Clinic's Clinical Core Laboratory Services, strongly suggests asking your local physician to send all reports, tests, studies, even biopsy slides and/or samples ahead of your visit. "Send everything," he advises, "because even though you may be coming for a urology consult, the human body is interconnected." A Mayo pathologist will review the pathology material, which might avoid the need for another biopsy.

## 2. Your Medications

Bring a list of your current medications and all dietary supplements, identified by their name and dosage. You should continue to take your prescribed medications until told otherwise by a Mayo physician. Bring your containers of medications with you to Rochester. (You can write a list of your current medications on the chart in the back of this book.)

### Insider Tip

Dr. Robert Frye comments: "If I could wave a wand to address one thing, it would be to get an accurate accounting of what medicines the patient is taking.

Patients are asked to fill out a medical history and current medicine list, but it is not always accurate. For a physician, it's critically important to know this information to help us make the proper diagnosis."

3. Your Medical History

You will be asked to give a "medical history" to your Mayo physician and other medical personnel during your visit. If you are admitted to the hospital, you may be asked to give this history numerous times. It is a good idea to have with you a comprehensive account including dates of your prior illnesses, surgeries, major medical procedures, and a history of diseases in your family. (Use the page "My Medical History" in the back of this book.) Bring your local doctors' names and contact information.

4. Your Medical Insurance

Know your insurance. What kind do you have: HMO, PPO, supplemental, or secondary coverage? Is Mayo Clinic "in network" or "out of network"? Definitely check with your medical insurance policy and/or provider to review what will be covered and what will not; you do not want to be "surprised" once you get to Rochester. If need be, billing estimates can be provided to give you an estimate of costs for particular exams, tests, surgeries, treatments, etc. before you come to Mayo. If you are paying out of pocket, Mayo will require a pre-service deposit of the estimated amount of services you are anticipated to have scheduled. There are options for charity care.

## 5. Who Needs to Go With You

*Bring at least one family member or friend with you to Rochester, if possible.* Mayo Clinic is an overwhelming place to navigate, especially by yourself. Most patients come with at least one person to help them. A family member or friend can act as a travel agent and logistics coordinator, arranging lodging, finding places to eat, and transporting or accompanying the patient from appointment to appointment. Remember—you are a patient, and you may not be feeling well. You will do well to have an advocate with you in any health care setting, even at Mayo.

You will also be under some stress as you go through the process of testing, meeting with doctors, and searching out answers to your medical problems. Many patients report that they think they understand what the doctor said, but not really. You need another set of ears. You will need physical and emotional support, especially if you are receiving difficult news. There will likely be long periods of waiting. Don't go it alone.

If you are coming to Mayo for surgery, you may want to have at least two people come with you. It is difficult to be in Rochester alone when someone is in the hospital; two people will offer much-needed support and companionship for each other while the patient recuperates.

### Insider Tip

Don Greenberg came to Mayo for treatment with his wife Nancy and adult children Robert Greenberg and Wendy Goldberg. Wendy brought along her laptop computer to log every single question, answer, instruction, appointment, and test result. In addition, at the end of your visit, or in your mail at home, you will usually receive a comprehensive report.

## 6. Your Pre-visit Packet

Once you have made your appointment, you will receive a packet of pre-visit information from the Clinic. This will often include:

Patient's Guide to Mayo Clinic
Fasting and other instructions for medical tests
Patient information
Appointment information
Lodging guide with calendar of events

## 7. Wheelchairs and Oxygen Tanks

If you are staying at a hotel connected to the Subway/Skyway system, you need not bring a wheelchair with you; they are in plentiful supply in and around the Clinic. Portable oxygen tanks are available from Mayo's Respiratory Care Office in the Eisenberg Building, Subway level, room Ei-S9. You don't need to drag your own around the campus. To request a portable oxygen tank, call 507-266-8758. This office is open Monday through Friday from 6:30 a.m. to 10:00 p.m. and closed on weekends and holidays. You can also call Mayo's General Services Department at 507-266-7100 to request an escort to that office. (These wonderful folks are available to assist patients in many ways; contact them by asking at any information desk or reception desk).

## Mayo Clinic Express Care

If you find yourself in Rochester and need care for common health concerns after the main Clinic appointment hours close at 5:00 p.m., the Mayo Clinic Express Care locations are an option. This service is available within two Hy-Vee grocery stores, one at 4221 West Circle Drive NW, one at 500 Crossroads Drive SW. Hours are Monday through Friday, 8:00 a.m. to 8:00 p.m., Saturday and Sunday, 9:00 a.m. to 5:00 p.m. Closed Thanksgiving, Christmas and New Year's Day; other holiday hours vary. You can make an appointment by logging onto Patient Online Services—www.mayoclinic.org/onlineservices—or simply walk-in and wait your turn.

# Chapter Three Your Journey to Rochester, Minnesota

## Insider Tip

THERE ARE AT LEAST TWELVE CITIES IN THE UNITED STATES CALLED "Rochester." Mayo Clinic is located in Minnesota—not Rochester, New York, Illinois, Kentucky, Indiana, Massachusetts, Ohio, Michigan, New Hampshire, Pennsylvania, Vermont, Washington or Wisconsin! You want Rochester, MINNESOTA.

## 1. By Car

Rochester (Minnesota!) is easily accessible by car.

### Traveling from the South:

Take Interstate 35 north to Interstate 90 east. Go north on U.S. Highway 63. At the city limits U.S. Highway 63 becomes Broadway and will take you directly into downtown Rochester.

### Traveling from the North:

Take Interstate 35 to U.S. Highway 14 east. Exit 2nd Street off ramp. Go north on 2nd Street past Saint Marys Hospital to Mayo Clinic buildings.

From the Minneapolis/St. Paul area:

Take U.S. Highway 52 south to Rochester. Exit Civic Center Drive. Go east to 4th Avenue.

Or—

Exit 2nd Street, travel past Saint Marys Hospital to the Mayo Clinic Buildings.

Traveling from the West:

Take U.S. Highway 14 (directly to Rochester) or Interstate 90 east, then U.S. 63 north.

Traveling from the East:

Take Interstate 90 west, then U.S. 63 north.

Or—

U.S. 14 west (directly to Rochester).

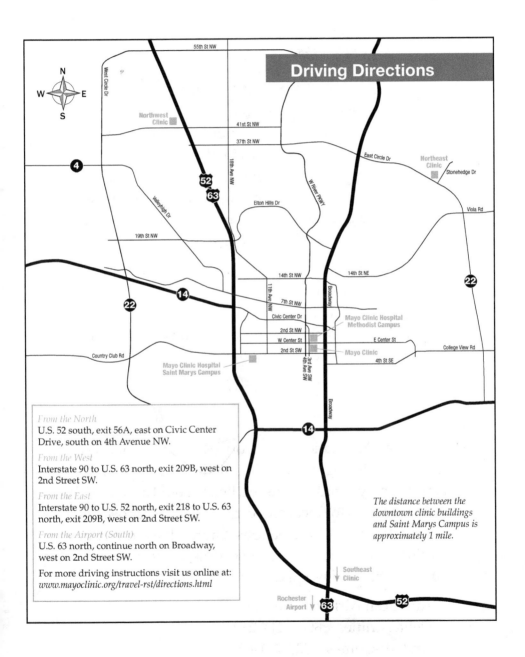

## Driving Directions

*From the North*
U.S. 52 south, exit 56A, east on Civic Center Drive, south on 4th Avenue NW.

*From the West*
Interstate 90 to U.S. 63 north, exit 209B, west on 2nd Street SW.

*From the East*
Interstate 90 to U.S. 52 north, exit 218 to U.S. 63 north, exit 209B, west on 2nd Street SW.

*From the Airport (South)*
U.S. 63 north, continue north on Broadway, west on 2nd Street SW.

For more driving instructions visit us online at:
*www.mayoclinic.org/travel-rst/directions.html*

*The distance between the downtown clinic buildings and Saint Marys Campus is approximately 1 mile.*

## Insider Tip

One of your biggest decisions before coming to Rochester is whether or not you want a car during your visit. The biggest advantage to having a car is freedom of mobility when you are not at the Clinic. On the other hand, parking in and around the downtown Mayo campus is limited and will cost you money — although Mayo operates several low-cost "parking ramps." Buses, taxis, Uber and Lyft are also available if you decide against bringing a car. Most of the off-campus hotels/motels offer free parking, and many of them provide free shuttle van service to the Clinic and Saint Marys Hospital.

On the other hand, there are at least ten hotels/motels that are directly connected to the Mayo buildings through the downtown Subway/Skyway system. If you choose one of these lodging facilities, you will not need a car to get to your appointments.

## 2. By Plane

Rochester International Airport (RST) is a small regional facility with regularly scheduled service provided by American Airlines, Delta Airlines, and United Airlines. American flies to Rochester direct from Chicago. Delta flies from Atlanta and Minneapolis. United flies from Chicago. Airlines often change their schedules. Check to see if the airlines offer a Mayo patient discount fare.

American Airlines   800-433-7300
Delta Airlines   800-221-1212
United Airlines   833-781-6301

## Insider Tip

Be sure to check with the airline to determine if your flight will necessitate climbing stairs to board, either at your point of departure or at Rochester International Airport. Not all of the six gates in Rochester have jetways, although they can provide for wheelchair-bound passengers to disembark.

There is a Mayo Clinic Information Desk located in the lobby of the Rochester airport.

Monday—Friday 6:30 a.m. to 10:30 p.m.
Saturday 10:00 a.m. to 6:00 p.m.
Sunday 2:45 p.m. to 10:45 p.m.
Closed Christmas and New Year's Day

You will find a selection of brochures about Mayo and the Mayo representative can assist with wheelchairs and transportation options.

## Insider Tip

These are the questions asked most often by Mayo patients arriving at the airport:

1. How far is the Clinic from the airport? (About twenty minutes by car.)

2. Where can I stay? (You can get a lodging brochure, but the Mayo staff is prohibited from endorsing any specific place.)

3. Can you help me with a wheelchair? (Wheelchairs are available.)

4. Can you provide an interpreter? (Mayo has a staff of interpreters available to translate for foreign visitors.)

5. Where do we go for appointments? (The Mayo buildings downtown.)

6. Where are the information desks? (In the lobby and Subway of the Gonda and Mayo Buildings)

7. What if I don't have an appointment? (You will be instructed as detailed above.)

8. How can I get in faster? (There is no magic answer to this question.)

Rochester International Airport also accommodates private aircraft and air ambulance services. A U.S. Customs Agent meets international flights arriving in Rochester.

3. Mayo Medical Transport

If a patient requires immediate air transportation by air ambulance or helicopter, Mayo Medical Transport can provide for your needs with one phone call to 800-237-6822 or 507-255-2808.

*Mayo MedAir* is a Mayo-staffed jet air ambulance that is essentially a mobile intensive care unit. Two pilots, a flight nurse and paramedic, and/or physicians, respiratory therapist and pediatric or neonatal intensive care nurses are assigned to the crew depending on the nature of the patient's needs. *Mayo One* is an emergency helicopter for transporting patients to and from Mayo Clinic and other medical centers or home after treatment. *Gold Cross* ground ambulance (800-237-6822) is operated by Mayo Medical Transport and provides transportation to and between medical facilities.

4. By Rail

There is daily Amtrak rail service (800-872-7245 or 507-452-8612) between Minneapolis and Chicago with a stop in Winona, Minnesota, forty-three miles east of Rochester. From Winona, ground transport can be arranged via taxi, limousine or commercial bus.

5. By Bus

Jefferson Bus Lines (507-282-6023) offers bus service to and around Rochester. Pick up a current schedule at the information desks in the Clinic.

## Getting from the Airport to the Clinic

The Rochester International Airport is located approximately fifteen miles south of downtown Rochester, just off U.S. Highway 63. You must arrange transportation from the airport to your hotel and/or the Clinic buildings. Here are some choices:

1. Taxi or Shuttle

Med City Taxi and Shuttle Service

Taxi Services, Shared Shuttle Service and Private Car Service

- Please call 507-282-8294 for more information
- Book a cab online

Total Transportation Shared Shuttle Service and Private Car Service
- Please call 507-322-5055 for more information
- https://totallimo.com

Yellow Cab   507-282-2222

GO Airport Shuttle   844-787-1670

Groome Transportation   507-280-9270

Groome (Go Carefree Shuttle)   888-781-5181 (toll-free)

Star Transportation   507-281-0969

### Ride Share Services

Ride share services such as Lyft and Uber are permitted to operate at RST. A designated ride share services pickup area is marked by signage on the sidewalk in front of the Terminal. Access to the pickup location is closest to the Ticketing doors. Ride share service companies are also permitted to drop-off passengers at their requested location at RST.

### Hotel Shuttles

Several area hotels offer shuttle service to and from the Rochester International Airport. Some hotel properties offer a free airport shuttle while others may charge a fee. It is best to contact your hotel in advance to ask about available shuttle services or to reserve a pick-up upon landing.

### Specialized Transportation

Total Transportation   651-770-5668 or https://totallimo.com

Handi Van of Rochester   507-281-3600—medical transport

Gold Cross (Mayo Clinic Ambulance)   507-225-2808

Land to Air EXPRESS

- Daily scheduled bus service to RST from: Mankato, Albert Lea, Austin, Owatonna, Waseca and Dodge Center.
- Please call 507-625-3977 or visit landtoairexpress.com

## Really Big Insider Tip

If you are coming to Rochester with at least one other person—and almost everyone does!—it will cost about the same amount of money to take a taxi to your hotel or the Clinic as it will to pay for two fares on the shuttle. You go directly where you want to go without having to endure the various shuttle stops to let other passengers off at their hotels.

## 2. Limousine

Several companies operate limousines that serve Rochester. *The big advantage of using the limousine service is that you can order the car ahead of time, and it will be waiting for you when your plane arrives.* Each company has different types of cars ranging from Lincoln Town Cars to stretch limos. Prices are competitive between the companies, although ask if the price includes tip or any other expenses. Here are the numbers for the limousine services:

Star Limousine (toll free: 866-440-2907, phone: 507-281-0969, or, email reservations@limostar.com; www.limostar.com

Gold Crown Limousine Service   507-285-9528

Med City Limousines   507-398-6659

Rochester Limo   507-322-3060

Chamberlain   507-208-1051

Corporate Car and Coach   507-261-4660

3. Rental Car

Several of the major rental car agencies have desks at the Rochester airport. Use their online booking services or 800 phone numbers to reserve a car at the best price. Look into a weekly rate, especially if you believe you'll be at the Clinic for five days or more.

## Flying into Minneapolis/St. Paul

Many Mayo patients find that air service to Minneapolis/St. Paul airport offers more choice and sometimes less expensive fares than flying directly to Rochester. The question then becomes: How do you get from Minneapolis/St. Paul to Rochester?

Go Rochester Direct (507-280-9270 or www.gorochesterdirect.com) operates a shuttle van service directly from the Minneapolis/ St. Paul International Airport to Rochester (with stops at most hotels) with more than ten departures daily between 7:00 a.m. and 10:15 p.m. Call for exact times and pickup location. Reservations are advised.

Rochester Shuttle Service (507-216-6354) is another option. rochestershuttleservice.com

Jefferson Bus Lines (800-231-2222 or 507-289-4037) also offers service from Minneapolis/St. Paul.

Go Rochester Direct (507-280-9270)

## Getting Around in Rochester

### Shuttle Service

With thousands of patients arriving at the Mayo downtown campus each day, an elaborate system of shuttle vans has developed to facilitate this large-scale movement of human beings.

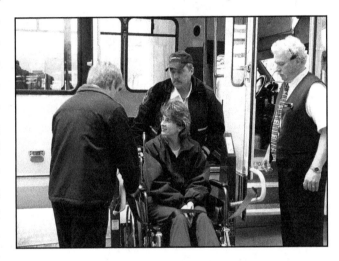

Mayo Clinic operates a free shuttle service for patients and visitors that runs continuously between the west door of the Gonda Building and the main entrance of Saint Marys Hospital— Mary Brigh Building from 6:45 a.m. to 5:30 p.m., Monday through Friday on days the Clinic is open. These shuttle vans are wheelchair-accessible. The shuttle begins its run at the Gonda Building at 6:45 a.m. The last shuttle from Saint Marys leaves at 5:15 p.m.

### Insider Tip

If you are scheduled for surgery and asked to arrive before 6:45 a.m., you will need to make other arrangements to get to the hospital; there is no Mayo patient shuttle running that early.

Most of the hotels provide free shuttle vans from their properties to the downtown Clinic buildings, dropping off at the Gonda Building main entrance on Third Avenue SW. Some hotels operate their own vans; most utilize the shuttle service operated by RST. For those requiring wheelchair-capable vans, contact R & S Transport (507-289-1988), Gold Cross (800-237-6822), or Yellow Cab (507-282-2222).

> ### Insider Tip
>
> Some hotels, Hilton Rochester Mayo Clinic Area and the Doubletree Hotel for example, offer an "on-demand" shuttle service that will take hotel guests anywhere they wish to go in Rochester at any time they want to go for free or a small fee.

## Bus

Rochester City Lines offers public bus service within Rochester and to outlying areas. Schedule and rate information is available at the information desks.

## Parking

Parking is a challenge in and around the Mayo buildings. Street parking is expensive and extremely time-limited. Downtown, the Clinic itself provides three parking "ramps," as these structures are called in Rochester, and one parking lot for patients:

Damon Parking Ramp, Third Avenue S.W. and First Street S.W.

Baldwin Parking Ramp, Fourth Avenue S.W., one block south of Second Street S.W.

Graham Parking Ramp, Third Avenue N.W. between First and Second Streets N.W.

Parking rates are reasonable at the Mayo-owned facilities. If you know you will be at the Clinic for more than three days, you can save money by purchasing a multiple-day parking pass. The pass is stamped with each use and does not expire.

## Insider Tip

The Damon Parking Ramp is the closest parking facility to the main entrance of the Gonda Building. The Graham Parking Ramp is opposite the buildings of the Methodist Hospital. The Baldwin Parking Ramp is the farthest away from the main buildings. The Damon and Graham parking ramps have two sides to them, one heading up and the other heading down toward the exit. Here's a great tip: In the early morning you can usually find parking on the "down" ramp. Cut over toward the exit on Level 4.

There are additional public parking ramps in the downtown area, and most of the major hotels offer parking, although their daily rates can be steep.

Valet parking is offered for a fee from 6:00 a.m. to 9:00 p.m. Monday through Friday at:

Saint Marys Campus—Mary Brigh Building, west entrance and Emergency Department

Mayo Clinic Downtown Campus, Charlton Building, west entrance.

For those arriving at the Gonda Building for appointments, valet parking is available from 6:00 a.m. to 6:00 p.m. Monday through Friday. Multiple-use discounted valet passes are available from parking attendants. For more information, call 507-293-3500.

## Accommodations— Where Should We Stay?

*The single most important decision affecting the quality of your stay in Rochester will be your choice of lodging.* In addition to the usual factors—price, amenities, restaurants—the location of the lodging will shape your experience more than anything.

Here's what you need to know.

Most lodging in Rochester is found in one of four areas:

> Downtown Area—near Mayo Clinic outpatient buildings and Rochester Methodist Hospital

> Saint Marys Area—across the street from the hospital

> Broadway Corridor—along Broadway (U.S. Highway 63) heading south toward the airport

> Airport—near the Rochester International Airport

Each area has its appeal.

### Downtown Area

The greatest advantage of staying in lodging downtown is *convenience.* If your hotel is connected to the Subway/Skyway system, you need never walk outside to get to your appointments in any Mayo Clinic outpatient buildings, to Rochester Methodist Hospital, or to shopping and eating areas. The closest lodging to the Gonda and Mayo Buildings is directly across the street and a short walk through the Subway corridors. You can literally leave your hotel room and be at your appointment in a matter of minutes. In fact, at some hotels a bellman will take you by wheelchair from your room to your appointment desk. This proximity also enables you to go back to your room for a rest between appointments.

The second advantage of the downtown hotels is that you are not dependent on a car or a shuttle to get you to your appointments. Parking can be a hassle during busy periods, and waiting for shuttles can be frustrating, especially if you are anxious to get back to your room.

A third advantage to staying downtown is that you are downtown, surrounded by good shopping, good restaurants, and safe streets. Rochester is a small (but growing) town, and the downtown is a safe area to walk around, even at night.

These advantages often come at a higher cost per night for a hotel room. Although there is a range of price points for these downtown hotels, typically the truly budget hotels are located along the Broadway corridor. If you have a car, you will also pay a daily parking rate to garage it at the hotel.

## Insider Tip

If you decide to lodge downtown, stay at one of the hotels that is connected to the Subway/Skyway system. The climate-controlled Subway/Skyway corridors enable you to get to your appointments, eating establishments, and stores regardless of the weather. As of this writing, the ten hotels connected to the Subway/Skyway system are: Hilton Rochester Mayo Clinic Area, Doubletree by Hilton Rochester-Mayo Clinic Area, Hilton Garden Inn, Brentwood Inn and Suites, Broadway Plaza, Kahler Grand Hotel, Kahler Inn and Suites, Residence Inn Rochester Mayo Clinic Area, Rochester Marriott Mayo Clinic Area, The Towers at Kahler Grand.

Insider Tip

For those seeking luxury accommodations, the newest lodging in Rochester is the Hilton Rochester Mayo Clinic Area which features spacious rooms and suites, including "The 19th Floor" featuring three spectacular Presidential Suites and four Governor's Suites, a large Executive Lounge, and a fleet of limousines providing on-demand rides to the Clinic buildings and around town. The Towers at Kahler Grand, a "hotel-within-a-hotel" on the top floor, directly across the street from the Mayo and Gonda Buildings. The Mayo Clinic itself is planning to build a five-star hotel on the top floors of the next addition of ten floors to the Gonda Building providing the closest access to the Clinic . . . just an elevator ride!

## Saint Marys Hospital Area

If you are admitted to Saint Marys Hospital, your family members may want to stay close by in one of the several lodging facilities directly across the street. Unfortunately, there are no underground Subway corridors connecting these hotels to the hospital. In inclement weather you can always take a shuttle to the front door of Saint Marys. Otherwise, having family members literally across the street offers them ease of access and you comfort of mind. There are some restaurants along Second Street S.W., but there are clearly more options downtown or on the Broadway corridor.

Insider Tip

You may have chosen to stay in a downtown hotel at the beginning of your Mayo experience, but then you are admitted to Saint Marys. Savvy family members will check out of the downtown hotel and move to a lodging option near the hospital. If you have a car, this will save you parking charges, since all the Saint Marys area hotels offer free parking for guests. Plus your family will be right across the street.

## Broadway Corridor

A number of lodging options, many of them offering budget rates, are located along Broadway (U.S. Highway 63). Nearly all of these hotel/motels offer shuttle service to the Mayo buildings.

## Airport

Americinn Rochester is the closest hotel to RST.

## Campgrounds

There are several campgrounds and RV parks in Rochester; check out the list on www.experiencerochestermn.com.

## Special Needs Lodging

These facilities are especially designed for patients with special medical needs:

Gift of Life Transplant House
705 2nd Street SW    507-288-7470
Organ transplant patients may qualify for a stay here.

Sandra J. Schulze American Cancer Society Hope Lodge
411 2nd Street NW    507-529-4673
For radiation and/or chemotherapy patients receiving treatment at Mayo Clinic.

Ronald McDonald House
850 2nd Street SW    507-282-3955
For families with children under age 18.

## Private Homes

If you prefer to stay in a private home, many options are found on VRBO and AirBnB.

A complete up-to-date list of lodging options can be found at www.experiencerochestermn.com.

# Questions to Ask

When searching for a place to stay, you might ask these important questions:

1. Is the property connected to the Subway/Skyway system?
2. Is there shuttle service from the front door of the property? (*Note: Some of the properties near Saint Marys Hospital ask guests to take the Mayo shuttle between the hospital and the downtown campus, necessitating a walk over to the hospital.*)
3. Are there long-term stay rates?
4. Is there a restaurant on site?
5. Is breakfast included?
6. Are pets allowed?
7. Is there an exercise room/swimming pool?
8. Is there high-speed Internet access?
9. Is a kitchenette unit available? A refrigerator?
10. Are there laundry facilities?
11. Which properties are "family-friendly"?
12. Are there movies on demand or premium cable channels in the room?

The Rochester Visitors and Convention is now called "Experience Rochester MN", website: experiencerochestermn.com (507-288-4331). Here you may find a lodging guide detailing all the accommodations available in Rochester. In 2020, there were 53 hotels/motels/guest houses, 3 extended stay lodging properties, and 4campgrounds/RV parks. This quarterly guide is sent to new Mayo patients in the pre-visit kit. The guide does not evaluate the property; it does, however, give a range of room rates, list amenities such as shuttle service to the Clinic, pool, health club, accessibility for the disabled, and include a few comments about the place.

## Insider Tip

A terrific place to start your search for lodging, advice on dining, and suggestions for things to do is ExperienceRochester, located in the Civic Center, 30 Civic Center Drive SE, Suite 200, Rochester, MN 55904, (phone 507-288-4331). They can help you narrow your choices and make good decisions about your stay in the area. Ask for the Lodging Guide.

## Insider Tip

There are few sources for ratings or reviews of accommodations in Rochester. Mayo Clinic does not endorse any lodging or eating establishment as a matter of policy, although you can ask the Patient Service Representatives or ask to be connected to the Concierge Desk; the good people there will help you sort out the alternatives once you describe your needs. The Automobile Association of America (AAA) does offer a rating of Rochester hotels/motels in their Minnesota Tour Book. On the Internet, TripAdvisor and Yelp have reviews of properties.

## Insider Tip

Many of the lodging properties offer a discount if your stay extends a week or longer. Ask. If you stay thirty days or longer in Rochester, you don't pay 11% lodging tax. You can also ask for discounts on hotel stays, dining, and shopping by showing your Mayo Clinic appointment itinerary, AAA card or AARP card and by looking in the local newspaper and visitor guides for coupons.

# The Lodging Guide

## 2020 Accommodations

$ = Under $50   $$ = $51–100   $$$ = Over $100

◆ Indicates Connection to Skyway/Pedestrian Subway
■ Indicates Downtown Location
✚ Close to Saint Marys Hospital
☎ Mayo Clinic provides shuttle service from Saint Marys Hospital to Mayo Clinic (for patients only) Monday through Friday from 7:00 a.m. to 5:30 p.m.

| Name • Address • Web Site • Phone • Fax | Number of Rooms | Standard Double Rates | Courtesy Clinic Shuttle | Suites | Free Continental Breakfast | Kitchenette Rooms | On-Site Restaurant | Indoor Pool | Pets Allowed | Handicap Accessible | Guest Laundry | Fitness Center | Free In-Room High-Speed Internet | Comments (Δ = may not have full/private bath) |
|---|---|---|---|---|---|---|---|---|---|---|---|---|---|---|
| **Aspen Select** ✚ • 1215 2nd Street SW, aspenselectrochester.com • (800) 366-3451 • (507) 288-2671 | 52 | $$ | ✓ | | ✓ | | | | | ✓ | ✓ | ✓ | ✓ | Newly renovated. Luxury mattresses, free breakfast, Wi-Fi, new fitness room, free parking and more. Directly across from Saint Marys. |
| **Aspen Suites** ✚ • 1211 2nd Street SW, aspensuitesrochester.com • (877) 335-6752 • (507) 289-6600 | 82 | $$ | ✓ | ✓ | ✓ | | | ✓ | ✓ | ✓ | ✓ | ✓ | ✓ | All-suite hotel, complimentary deluxe breakfast, swimming pool and whirlpool, free garage parking, newly remodeled. |
| **Centerstone Plaza Hotel Soldiers Field-Mayo Clinic Area** ■ • 401 6th Street SW • soldiersfield.com • (800) 366-2067 • (507) 288-2677 | 214 | $$ | ✓ | | | | ✓ | ✓ | ✓ | ✓ | ✓ | ✓ | ✓ | TripAdvisor Award of Excellence. Mayo Clinic/downtown/airport express shuttle. Free Wi-Fi, hot breakfast and gluten-free restaurant. |
| **Courtyard by Marriott Rochester/Saint Marys** ✚ • 161 13th Avenue SW, courtyardrochester.com • (800) 321-2211 • (507) 536-0040 | 117 | $$ | ✓ | ✓ | | ✓ | ✓ | ✓ | | ✓ | ✓ | ✓ | ✓ | Microwave/fridge in every room. Rooms with balconies. Jacuzzi suites. Across the street from Saint Marys. |
| **DoubleTree by Hilton Rochester - Mayo Clinic Area** ◆ ■ • 150 S Broadway • rochesterdowntown.doubletree.com • (507) 281-8000 | 212 | $$$ | ✓ | ✓ | | ✓ | ✓ | ✓ | | ✓ | ✓ | ✓ | ✓ | Skyway and town car service to Mayo Clinic, mall, restaurants. Microwave/fridge in every room. Complimentary Wi-Fi, 100 percent smoke free. |
| **Fairfield Inn & Suites** • 470 17th Avenue NW, marriott.com/rstfi • (844) 368-5209 • (507) 258-7300 | 91 | $$ | ✓ | ✓ | ✓ | | | ✓ | | ✓ | ✓ | ✓ | ✓ | Located off of US 52, near Mayo Clinic and Saint Marys Hospital. Free parking, Wi-Fi and breakfast. Shuttle to Mayo Clinic and Saint Marys. |
| **Hilton Garden Inn Downtown Rochester** ◆ ■ • 225 S Broadway • rochestermn.hgi.com • (507) 285-1234 | 143 | $$ | ✓ | ✓ | | | ✓ | ✓ | ✓ | ✓ | ✓ | ✓ | ✓ | Skyway and town car service to Mayo Clinic and downtown, microwave/fridge in every room, complimentary Wi-Fi, 100 percent smoke free. |
| **Home2 Suites by Hilton Rochester Mayo Clinic Area** • 831 16th Street SW • rochestermayoclinicarea.home2suitesbyhilton.com/ • 1-800-gohiltons • (507) 361-4200 | 103 | $$ | ✓ | ✓ | ✓ | ✓ | | ✓ | | ✓ | ✓ | ✓ | ✓ | New all-suite hotel. Two miles to Mayo Clinic/Mayo Civic Center. Free secured underground parking/hot breakfast/internet/shuttle service to Mayo Clinic. Full kitchenette. |
| **Homewood Suites by Hilton** ✚ • 165 13th Avenue SW, hilton.com/en/hotels/rstrhw-homewoodsuites-rochester-mayo-clinic-area-saint-marys • (507) 218-3320 | 108 | $$ | ✓ | ✓ | ✓ | ✓ | | ✓ | ✓ | ✓ | ✓ | ✓ | ✓ | Upscale, extended stay hotel. All suites have separate living/sleeping areas, full kitchens and more. Hot, full breakfast. |
| **SpringHill Suites by Marriott** ✚ • 1125 2nd Street SW, springhillrochester.com • (800) 678-9894 • (507) 281-5455 | 86 | $ | ✓ | ✓ | ✓ | | | ✓ | | ✓ | ✓ | ✓ | ✓ | Directly across from Saint Marys Hospital, close to restaurants, three-star rating. |
| **2nd Street Inn & Suites** ✚ • 1013 2nd Street SW • rgilodging.com (507) 424-1170 | 44 | $ | ✓ | | ✓ | | | | | ✓ | ✓ | | ✓ | Near Saint Marys Hospital. Free parking. |
| **5th Avenue Inn & Suites** ■ • 20 5th Avenue NW rgilodging.com (877) 678-4837 • (507) 289-3987 | 62 | $ | ✓ | | ✓ | | | | | ✓ | ✓ | | ✓ | Free off-street parking. Recently renovated. Voicemail. Walking distance to Mayo Clinic. |

## 2020 Accommodations

$ = Under $50   $$ = $51–100   $$$ = Over $100
◆ Indicates Connection to Skyway/Pedestrian Subway
■ Indicates Downtown Location
✚ Close to Saint Marys Hospital
🚐 Mayo Clinic provides shuttle service from Saint Marys Hospital to Mayo Clinic (for patients only) Monday through Friday from 7:00 a.m. to 5:30 p.m.

Δ = may not have full/private bath

| Name • Address • Web Site • Phone • Fax | Number of Rooms | Standard Double Rates | Courtesy Clinic Shuttle | Suites | Free Continental Breakfast | Kitchenette Rooms | On-Site Restaurant | Indoor Pool | Pets Allowed | Handicap Accessible | Guest Laundry | Fitness Center | Free In-Room High-Speed Internet | Comments |
|---|---|---|---|---|---|---|---|---|---|---|---|---|---|---|
| **AmericInn Rochester** • 7320 Airport View Drive SW americinn.com • (800) 634-3444 • (507) 536-7000 | 72 | $$ | ✓ | ✓ | ✓ | | | ✓ | ✓ | ✓ | ✓ | ✓ | ✓ | Featuring 72 freshly remodeled rooms, hospitality suite, pool, hot tub, workout room, business center, hot continental breakfast. |
| **Apache Hotel** • 1517 16th Street SW apachehotel.com • (800) 552-7224 • (507) 289-8866 | 149 | $$ | ✓ | ✓ | ✓ | | ✓ | ✓ | ✓ | ✓ | ✓ | ✓ | ✓ | Water slide, toddler water park, free parking, across from Apache Mall. |
| **Best Price Inn** • 1817 S Broadway bestpriceinn.net • (800) 708-2376 • (507) 289-2376 | 18 | $ | | | ✓ | | | | | ✓ | | | ✓ | Microwave/fridge in every room. Walking distance to restaurants. Free parking. |
| **Brentwood Inn & Suites** ◆■ • 123 4th Avenue NW brentwoodinn.com • (800) 658-7045 • (507) 288-8011 | 93 | $$ | ✓ | ✓ | ✓ | | | | | ✓ | | | ✓ | Subway access to Mayo Clinic and shopping. Free off-street parking. Smoke free. Expanded continental breakfast. |
| **Broadway Plaza** ◆■ • 15 1st Street SE rochesterbroadwayplaza.com • (507) 424-4200 | 145 | $$$ | ✓ | ✓ | ✓ | ✓ | | ✓ | | ✓ | ✓ | ✓ | ✓ | Fully furnished 1-4 bedroom apartments. Full kitchens with washer/dryer. Located within walking distance to Mayo Clinic. |
| **Candlewood Suites** • 1640 S Broadway ihg.com/candlewood/hotels/us/en/rochester/rstcw/hoteldetail (507) 361-6000 | 77 | $$ | | ✓ | | ✓ | | | | ✓ | ✓ | ✓ | ✓ | New hotel with kitchens and recliners in every suite. Free laundry, heated underground parking and fitness center. Pet friendly. |
| **Comfort Inn & Suites** • 2005 Commerce Drive NW choicehotels.com/minnesota/rochester/comfort-inn-hotels/mn153 (800) 300-8800 • (507) 281-6850 | 84 | $$ | ✓ | ✓ | ✓ | | | ✓ | | ✓ | ✓ | ✓ | ✓ | Located in an upcoming area. Featuring hot complimentary breakfast and indoor pool. |
| **Comfort Suites** • 4141 Maine Avenue SE choicehotels.com/hotel/MN106 • (507) 424-2720 | 60 | $$ | ✓ | ✓ | ✓ | | | ✓ | | ✓ | ✓ | ✓ | ✓ | 100 percent smoke free, meeting room, near movie theater, restaurants, shopping. |
| **Country Inn & Suites By Carlson North** • 4323 Highway 52 N countryinns.com/rochestermn_north • (800) 456-4000 • (507) 285-3335 | 104 | $$ | ✓ | ✓ | ✓ | | | ✓ | | ✓ | ✓ | ✓ | ✓ | Weekday shuttle to Mayo, IBM and airport. Fridge and microwave in all rooms, guest laundry, exercise room, business center and free wireless internet access. |
| **Country Inn & Suites By Radisson** • Rochester South 77 Woodlake Drive SE • countryinns.com/clinic (800) 456-4000 • (507) 287-6758 | | $$ | ✓ | ✓ | ✓ | | | ✓ | ✓ | ✓ | ✓ | ✓ | ✓ | Enjoy TripAdvisor award-winning service, free hot breakfast daily, parking, clinic shuttle weekdays, wireless internet access and more. |
| **Days Inn & Suites South** • 3595 Commercial Drive SW daysinn.com • (507) 206-4675 | 117 | $ | ✓ | ✓ | ✓ | ✓ | | | | ✓ | ✓ | ✓ | ✓ | Full kitchens, onsite guest laundry, five miles from Mayo Clinic, free parking, cable and HBO. |
| **Econo Lodge by Choice Hotels** • 1850 S Broadway choicehotels.com/minnesota/rochester/econo-lodge-hotels/mn045?brand=EL(800) • 553-2666 • (507) 282-9905 | 62 | $ | ✓ | ✓ | ✓ | | | | | ✓ | | ✓ | ✓ | Award winning, family owned and operated, 100 percent smoke free, microwave/fridge, deluxe breakfast, free wireless, next to Perkins. |

## 2020 Accommodations

$ = Under $50    $$ = $51–100    $$$ = Over $100
♦ Indicates Connection to Skyway/Pedestrian Subway
■ Indicates Downtown Location
✛ Close to Saint Marys Hospital
✛* Mayo Clinic provides shuttle service from Saint Marys Hospital to Mayo Clinic (for patients only) Monday through Friday from 7:00 a.m. to 5:30 p.m.

| Name • Address • Web Site • Phone • Fax | Number of Rooms | Standard Double Rates | Courtesy Clinic Shuttle | Suites | Free Continental Breakfast | Kitchenette Rooms | On-Site Restaurant | Indoor Pool | Pets Allowed | Handicap Accessible | Guest Laundry | Fitness Center | Free In-Room High-Speed Internet | Comments (△ = may not have full/private bath) |
|---|---|---|---|---|---|---|---|---|---|---|---|---|---|---|
| Extended Stay America North • 2814 43rd Street NW extendedstayamerica.com • (800) 398-7829 • (507) 289-7444 | 95 | $ | | ✓ | | ✓ | | | | ✓ | ✓ | | ✓ | Recliners, extended cable TV, fully equipped kitchen, free local calls and voicemail. |
| Extended Stay America South • 55 Woodlake Drive SE extendedstayamerica.com • (800) 398-7829 • (507) 536-7444 | 98 | $ | | ✓ | | ✓ | | | ✓ | ✓ | ✓ | | ✓ | Recliners, extended cable TV, fully equipped kitchen, free local calls and voicemail. Free shuttle to the Mayo Clinic, weekly and monthly rates available. Pets allowed. |
| GuestHouse International Inn & Suites ✛ • 435 16th Avenue NW redlion.com/guesthouse/mn/rochester/guesthouse-rochester (877) 374-9090 • (507) 288-9090 | 118 | $ | ✓ | ✓ | ✓ | ✓ | | ✓ | | ✓ | ✓ | | ✓ | Newly remodeled pool area, 100 percent smoke free, microwave/fridge, free parking, special rates |
| Hampton Inn & Suites Rochester - North • 2870 59th Street NW rochesternorthsuites.hamptoninn.com • (507) 289-6100 | 124 | $$ | ✓ | ✓ | ✓ | | | ✓ | | ✓ | ✓ | ✓ | ✓ | Enjoy 124 rooms, 40 suites, free wireless and a free hot breakfast. |
| Hampton Inn • 1755 S Broadway rochestermn.hamptoninn.com • (800) 426-7866 • (507) 287-9050 | 103 | $$ | ✓ | ✓ | ✓ | | | ✓ | | ✓ | ✓ | ✓ | ✓ | Free high-speed wireless internet, free hot breakfast, free parking, HDTV, 100 percent smoke free. |
| Hilton Rochester Mayo Clinic Area ♦■ • 10 E Center Street rochestermayoclinicarea.hilton.com • (507) 258-5757 | 264 | $$$ | | ✓ | ✓ | | ✓ | ✓ | | ✓ | ✓ | ✓ | ✓ | Located two blocks from Mayo Clinic. Rooms/suites range from 390–1,600 square feet. Rooftop terrace, indoor pool and fitness center. |
| Holiday Inn Express & Suites ✛ • 155 16th Avenue SW hotelnearmayoclinicrochester.com • (507) 226-8700 | 85 | $$ | ✓ | ✓ | ✓ | | | ✓ | | ✓ | ✓ | ✓ | ✓ | Conveniently located next to US-52 and 2nd Street. Near Saint Marys Hospital. |
| Hotel Indigo ■ • 220 S Broadway ihg.com/hotelindigo/hotels/us/en/rochester • (507) 252-8200 | 173 | $$ | | | | | ✓ | | | ✓ | | ✓ | ✓ | To be completed in early 2020. To complete its luxury feel, amenities will include a pool, fitness center and rooftop bar. |
| Kahler Grand Hotel ♦■ • 20 2nd Avenue SW thekahlerhotel.com • (800) 533-1655 • (507) 280-6200 | 552 | $$ | ✓ | ✓ | | | ✓ | ✓ | | ✓ | ✓ | ✓ | ✓ | Closest full-service hotel directly connected to Mayo Clinic. Modest to luxurious accomodations. |
| Kahler Inn & Suites ■ • 9 3rd Avenue NW kahlerinnsuites.com • (800) 533-1655 • (507) 285-9200 | 271 | $$ | ✓ | ✓ | ✓ | | ✓ | ✓ | | ✓ | ✓ | ✓ | ✓ | Adjoins Mayo-pedestrian subway. Finest economy suites. Free breakfast. |
| La Quinta Inn & Suites • 4353 Canal Place SE laquintarochestermn.com • (800) 753-3757 • (507) 289-4200 | 83 | $$ | ✓ | ✓ | ✓ | | | ✓ | ✓ | ✓ | ✓ | ✓ | ✓ | Free hot buffet breakfast. Free Mayo Clinic/airport shuttle. Pools, spa, fridge, microwave, Keurig, 40-inch TV/DVD player. Top rated. |
| Mainstay Suites • 2109 Commerce Drive NW choicehotels.com/minnesota/rochester/mainstay-hotels/mn181 (507) 282-2576 | 41 | $$ | ✓ | ✓ | ✓ | ✓ | | ✓ | ✓ | ✓ | ✓ | ✓ | ✓ | Free Mayo shuttle, free hot breakfast, free parking, pool, Wi-Fi, fitness center. Full kitchens and pullout couches. Extended stay. |
| Maria's Room & Kitchenettes ✛ • 1139 2nd Street SW mariasroomsatmayo.com • (507) 208-5785 | 21 | $ | | | | ✓ | | | | ✓ | ✓ | | ✓ | Across from Saint Marys Hospital. Free parking. Microwave/fridge in every room. Coffee shop and restaurants are just steps away. |

## 2020 Accommodations

$ = Under $50    $$ = $51–100    $$$ = Over $100
◆ Indicates Connection to Skyway/Pedestrian Subway
■ Indicates Downtown Location
✛ Close to Saint Marys Hospital
📷* Mayo Clinic provides shuttle service from Saint Marys Hospital to Mayo Clinic (for patients only) Monday through Friday from 7:00 a.m. to 5:30 p.m.

| Name • Address • Web Site • Phone • Fax | Number of Rooms | Standard Double Rates | Courtesy Clinic Shuttle | Suites | Free Continental Breakfast | Kitchenette Rooms | On-Site Restaurant | Indoor Pool | Pets Allowed | Handicap Accessible | Guest Laundry | Fitness Center | Free In-Room High-Speed Internet | Comments (△ = may not have full/private bath) |
|---|---|---|---|---|---|---|---|---|---|---|---|---|---|---|
| **Microtel Inn & Suites North** • 4210 Highway 52 N microtelinn.com/hotels/minnesota/rochester/microtel-inn-and-suites-rochester/hotel-overview (800) 245-9535 • (507) 286-8780 | 81 | $ | ✓ | ✓ | ✓ | | | | | | ✓ | ✓ | | Free breakfast and free shuttle to Mayo. Free Wi-Fi and long distance phone calls. Fitness center, business center. 100 percent smoke free. |
| **Microtel Inn & Suites South** • 4165 Maine Avenue SE microtelinn.com • (800) 337-0050 • (507) 289-4900 | 88 | $ | ✓ | ✓ | ✓ | | | | | | ✓ | ✓ | | Free Mayo shuttle. Pool, fitness center, free hot buffet breakfast. HDTV, fridge, microwave, coffee maker. Award-winner. |
| **Motel 6** • 2107 W Frontage Road motel6.com • (800) 466-8356 • (507) 282-6625 | 86 | $ | ✓ | ✓ | ✓ | | | | | | ✓ | | | Free parking, outdoor pool, near restaurants and shopping. |
| **Quality Inn** • 5708 Bandel Road NW choicehotels.com/minnesota/rochester/quality-inn-hotels/mn087 (877) 424-6423 • (507) 289-3434 | 78 | $$ | ✓ | ✓ | ✓ | | | | | ✓ | ✓ | | | Complimentary enhanced breakfast. Mayo Clinic rates, Corp., AARP rates. Meeting room. |
| **Quality Inn & Suites** • 1620 1st Avenue SE choicehotels.com/minnesota/rochester/quality-inn-hotels/mn421 (800) 544-2717 • (507) 282-8091 | 41 | $ | ✓ | ✓ | ✓ | ✓ | | | | ✓ | | | | Two-room suites with fully furnished kitchenettes. Complimentary transportation to Mayo Clinic. Free parking. |
| **Rainbow Inn** ✛ • 1217 2nd Street SW (507) 288-0025 | 12 | $ | | | | ✓ | | | | ✓ | | | | Directly across from Saint Marys main door. |
| **Ramada by Wyndham Rochester Mayo Clinic Area** 1625 S Broadway • wyndhamhotels.com • (507) 328-0217 | 145 | $ | ✓ | ✓ | ✓ | ✓ | ✓ | ✓ | ✓ | ✓ | ✓ | | | Newly remodeled. Microwave/fridge in all rooms. |
| **Red Carpet Inn** • 2214 S Broadway • rochester.redcarpetinnhotels.com (800) 658-7048 • (507) 282-7448 | 30 | $ | | | | | | | ✓ | ✓ | | | | All rooms with microwave/fridge, some with recliners. Free local calls and parking. 100 percent smoke free. |
| **Residence Inn Rochester Mayo Clinic Area** ◆■ • 441 W Center Street marriott.com/rstri/ • (877) 623-7775 • (507) 292-1400 | 89 | $$ | ✓ | ✓ | ✓ | ✓ | | ✓ | ✓ | ✓ | ✓ | ✓ | | Take advantage of free internet, grocery service and connection to Mayo Clinic. |
| **Rochester Inn** • 1837 S Broadway rochesterinnmn.com • (800) 890-3871 • (507) 288-2031 | 22 | $ | | | | | | | | | | | | Restaurants nearby, family owned, free parking, first-level units and free coffee. |
| **Rochester Marriott Mayo Clinic Area** ◆■ • 101 1st Avenue SW marriott.com/rstmc/ • (877) 623-7775 • (507) 280-6000 | 202 | $$$ | ✓ | ✓ | | | ✓ | ✓ | | ✓ | ✓ | ✓ | | Directly connected to Mayo Clinic. Rochester's premier full-service hotel. Marriott Rewards. |
| **Sleep Inn** • 2109 Commerce Drive NW choicehotels.com/minnesota/rochester/sleep-inn-hotels/mn180 (507) 282-2364 | 40 | $$ | ✓ | ✓ | ✓ | | | ✓ | | ✓ | ✓ | ✓ | | Free Mayo shuttle, free hot breakfast, free parking, pool, Wi-Fi, fitness center. Features modern decor, microwave, fridge, 43-inch TV. |
| **Super 8 by Wyndham Fairgrounds Area** • 1230 S Broadway wyndhamhotels.com/super-8/rochesterminnesota/super-8-rochester-fairgrounds-area/overview • (800) 800-8000 • (507) 288-8288 | 87 | $ | ✓ | ✓ | ✓ | | ✓ | ✓ | ✓ | ✓ | ✓ | ✓ | | Adjacent to Denny's Restaurant. Indoor pool. Free parking. |

## 2020 Accommodations

$ = Under $50   $$ = $51–100   $$$ = Over $100
♦ Indicates Connection to Skyway/Pedestrain Subway
■ Indicates Downtown Location
✚ Close to Saint Marys Hospital
📱* Mayo Clinic provides shuttle service from Saint Marys Hospital to Mayo Clinic (for patients only) Monday through Friday from 7:00 a.m. to 5:30 p.m.

△ = may not have full/private bath

| Name • Address • Web Site • Phone • Fax | Number of Rooms | Standard Double Rates | Comments |
|---|---|---|---|
| Super 8 S Broadway • 106 21st Street SE<br>wyndhamhotels.com/super-8/rochesterminnesota/super-8-rochester-south-broadway/overview • (507) 282-1756 | 73 | $ | All rooms with microwave/fridge. Clinic, AARP rates. |
| The Towers at Kahler Grand ♦✚ • 20 2nd Avenue SW<br>towersatkahlergrand.com • (507) 208-1409 | 44 | $$$ | Rochester's only luxury hotel with fivestar amenities. |
| TownePlace Suites by Marriott • 2829 43rd Street NW<br>marriott.com/hotels/travel/rsttstowneplace-suites-rochester (866) 814-1200 • (507) 281-1200 | 82 | $$ | All-suite hotel. Corporate and medical rates available. Indoor water park. 100 percent smoke free. |

## Extended Stay Housing

**Annie's Patient Hospitality House • 3611 18th Avenue NW**
(507) 273-0470 • shnrochestermn.com/housing/annie-s-patient-hospitality-house.php
1-2 bedroom furnished apartments. Full kitchens, laundry, parking, cable/phone/high-speed internet included.

**Centerstone Plaza Hotel Soldiers Field - Mayo Clinic Area • 401 6th Street SW**
(800) 366-2067, (507) 288-2677 • soldiersfield.com
TripAdvisor Award of Excellence. Mayo Clinic/downtown/airport express shuttle. Free Wi-Fi, hot breakfast and gluten free restaurant.

**Serenity House Network Medical Lodging • 2041 31st Place NW**
(507) 273-0470 • shnrochestermn.com
Licensed medical lodging. 1-3 bedroom furnished patient apartments and homes. Full kitchens, free laundry. Near Mayo Clinic.

**Hyatt House • 315 First Avenue NW**
hyatt.com/brands/hyatt-house
Opening in late summer 2020, this extended stay hotel will feature 173 rooms, located conveniently on the northern side of downtown Rochester near Mayo Clinic.

**The Kathy House • 1414 Pahama Court NW • (507) 261-4104 • shawnburyska.com/kathyhouse/**
Extensively remodeled 3 bedroom and 2 bathroom home near Mayo Clinic featuring many amenities.

## Campgrounds/RV Parks   *Call ahead for availability*

**AutumnWoods RV Park • 1067 Autumnwoods Circle SW**
(866) 397-8489, (507) 990-2983 • autumnwoodsrvpark.com
93 full hook sites, clean showers and restroom facilities, laundry, security and Wi-Fi. Open seasonally.

**Bob's Trailer Court & RV Parking • 1915 Marion Road SE • (507) 272-9512**
Year-round. Full hook-ups. Call ahead for availability.

**Ferguson's Willow Creek Campground & RV Park • 5525 Highway 63 S**
(507) 281-0304 • willowcreeksite.com
50 sites, full and partial hook-ups, showers, partially wooded area.

**Rochester KOA • 5232 65th Avenue SE • (800) 562-5232, (507) 288-0785 • rochesterkoa.com**
73 sites, full and partial hook-ups, showers, laundry, recreation, pool, store, small playground.

# Chapter Four Navigating The Clinic

## How Not to Be Intimidated by the Enormity of It All

THE FIRST DAY AT MAYO CLINIC CAN BE AN OVERWHELMING EXPERIENCE. The downtown campus spans twelve city blocks. The buildings are connected by a maze of Subway and Skyway corridors that take some navigating skills. There is a unique system of appointments to figure out and instructions to follow. The physicians and allied health professionals have differentiated roles and titles. People talk in "Mayo-ese," an entire language of terms and names unfamiliar to the newcomer. Some of the elevators in the Mayo and Gonda Buildings go from the Subway to the 10th floor, while another bank of elevators goes higher. The directional signs are very good, but many people find themselves disoriented and need to ask for help finding the location of their next appointment.

The good folks at Mayo know all this. They are committed to making the Mayo experience as smooth and pleasant as possible. There is a "Way-Finding Committee" whose only task is to find better ways to help people get around the campus. There is a whole area of patient communications charged with explaining the Mayo system. There is a host of professionals and volunteers who are positioned to assist patients and family members with directions, information, advice, escort services, and a comforting word of welcome.

*The best way to experience Mayo is to be unafraid to ask questions, to ask for assistance, to ask for help.* Every single employee of Mayo—from the CEO to the cafeteria server—is given training in the fine art of caring. Anyone wearing a blue Mayo name tag is encouraged to look out for people who look lost, to offer help, to guide you to your next appointment.

It is also helpful to read carefully all the information sent to you *before* arriving in Rochester. Fill out the Patient Survey, review your medical history, create a list of medications, assemble or send your X rays and reports, write down your questions.

When you arrive in Rochester, come to the Clinic early so you are not rushed to find your first appointment location. Get your bearings—the next sections of the *Insider's Guide* will help you with this. Trust that it will get easier to find your way around, to negotiate the Mayo system, to explore the Subway, to locate a place to eat, to sit down and rest.

### Insider Tip

To better orient yourself to Subway/Skyway system, take the "Subway/Skyway System" map in Appendix 2 and walk through to the Clinic the night before you need to go to an appointment. Go in the evening (before 7:00 p.m. if you want to access Clinic buildings) when Subways are quiet. Trace the route from your hotel. Notice landmarks along the way. Notice the directional signs. You'll find that after doing the route once or twice you will feel more confident.

You have chosen to become a patient at one of the greatest medical centers in the history of humankind. You are in great hands—healing hands with only one goal: your good health.

# Your First Day

## ARRIVING AT THE CLINIC

### By Car

If you drive to the downtown Clinic campus, you will most likely park in one of the major Clinic-operated multi-level parking ramps. If you are coming for appointments in the central complex of Gonda/Mayo Buildings, park in the largest ramp, the *Damon Parking Ramp* (3rd Avenue S.W. and 1st Street S.W.), located directly across from the main entrance of the Gonda Building. Note where you parked and take the elevator to the Subway Level. As you exit the elevator proceed straight ahead (notice the interesting photographic mural "My Brother and I" detailing the timeline of the Mayo brothers' development of the Clinic, and look above to marvel at the Chihuly chandeliers) and turn right at the Geffen Auditorium to reach the Gonda/Mayo elevator bank.

> ### Insider Tip
>
> When the Damon Parking Ramp is full, as it often is after 9:00 a.m. on most weekdays, you will be directed to the Graham Parking Ramp, two blocks ahead on 3rd Avenue.

If you are headed to the Rochester Methodist Hospital, park in the Graham Parking Ramp (3rd Avenue N.W. between 1st and

2nd Street N.W.), take the elevator to the Subway Level, and enter through the Charlton North Building.

If you have a first appointment in the Baldwin Building, you may choose to park in the Baldwin Parking Ramp (4th Avenue S.W., one block south of 2nd Street S.W.).

There are other parking ramps operated by the City of Rochester and local hotels. Parking on the street is highly restricted and metered.

### Insider Tip

You will be much better off not parking on the street. The time allowed at each meter is limited, and you will need to worry about feeding the meter throughout the day, requiring you to run back and forth between your appointments. The Mayo-operated parking ramps are your best bet, followed by the city-operated ramps.

## Valet Parking

Valet parking is available for a fee at Gonda Building, west entrance, Monday through Friday, 6:00 a.m. to 6:00 p.m.; Charlton Building, west entrance, Monday through Friday, 6:00 a.m. to 9:00 p.m., Saint Marys Mary Brigh Building and Saint Marys Emergency Department, Monday through Friday, 6:00 a.m. to 9:00 p.m. Multiple use discounted valet parking passes are available from parking attendants or at most Information Desks and do not expire.

## Disabled Parking

There are a number of parking spaces designated for disabled access on each floor of the Mayo-operated parking ramps, located right next to the entrance for the elevators. These spaces are marked with the familiar blue sign featuring a wheelchair. Van-accessible and state disabled parking spaces are available in the Graham Parking Ramp. You will be charged the regular parking rate.

### Insider Tip

If you are driving to Rochester—or renting a car—and have a patient requiring wheelchair assistance, bring along your disabled parking permit and hang it from your rearview mirror. It will be honored, no matter which state issued the permit.

### Really Big Insider Tip

You may park free of charge at any city meter if you have a disabled parking permit.

## By Shuttle

Nearly every hotel and motel in Rochester offers a shuttle van service to bring patients and family members to the downtown campus. Some of these shuttles are operated by the hotel exclusively for its guests. RST operates a shuttle that picks up passengers at a number of hotels. All of the shuttles drop passengers at the main entrance of the Gonda Building. Some continue on to drop passengers at the Rochester Methodist Hospital (the Charlton West drop off) and at Saint Marys Hospital.

Once you are at the main downtown campus of the Clinic or at Saint Marys Hospital, you may take a Mayo Clinic-operated patient shuttle that runs continuously between the Gonda Building and Saint Marys Hospital from 6:45 a.m. to 5:30 p.m. (last departure from Saint Marys is at 5:15 p.m.) Monday through Friday. The van arrives and departs from the main entrance (west door) of the Gonda Building and the west entrance of Saint

Marys Hospital, Mary Brigh Building. There is a wheelchair-accessible lift on the vehicle.

## Wheelchairs/Walkers/Scooters

One of the truly amazing sights you first encounter at Mayo Clinic is the row upon row of wheelchairs stacked at the major entrances to the buildings, both at the outpatient buildings and at the hospitals. Mayo has anticipated the need for hundreds of wheelchairs—not just for disabled patients, but for anyone who does not feel well and needs assistance in navigating the distances between appointments. The wheelchairs are available free of charge. Walkers are also available. Ask a door attendant or any staff member at a reception desk to arrange this service, or call 507-266-7100. Return the wheelchair to an entrance such as the Gonda main entrance, or call 507-538-6100 to leave a message reporting where you left it. You may also rent a scooter from the Mayo Store (507-284-9669 or 1-888-303-9354).

### Insider Tip

There is no need to bring your own wheelchair to Rochester. Not only does the Clinic provide wheelchairs to use, but most hotels have wheelchairs available. There are stacks of wheelchairs at the airport. Many patients staying in downtown hotels borrow a Mayo wheelchair and keep it in the room. Mayo doesn't mind; they are mainly interested in your comfort and ease of transportation. Just don't take it home!

## Special Needs Accessibility

All patient care and public areas of the Mayo campus are accessible, as is much of downtown Rochester. Hotels, restaurants, and shops are sensitive to those with special needs. Wheel-chair-accessible restrooms are located in all Mayo buildings and marked as such. "Special needs restrooms" designed for a single patient and a helper are available on the Subway Level of the Mayo Building and on the main floor of the Joseph Building in Saint Marys Hospital.

Sign language interpreters may be requested on your registra-tion form or arranged by calling 507-284-2741. You can also ask to speak to a sign language interpreter at the Concierge Services desk just inside the International Center, Mayo Building, lobby level. TDD services for the deaf and volume-controlled tele-phones are located on the Subway Level of the Mayo Building.

## Escorts

If you need mobility assistance in getting around the Clinic, an escort from General Service can be called from the main entrance, information desk, or reception desk on campus. You may also call directly for an escort by contacting General Ser-vice Dispatch, 507-266-7100. In short order an escort will arrive at your location with a wheelchair and take you anywhere you need to go within the Clinic buildings. Escorts are quite knowl-edgeable about the Clinic and can give you directions or answer questions.

### Insider Tip

Several of the downtown hotels provide escort service from your room to appointments at the Clinic. Inquire at the front desk.

## Babies at Mayo

Strollers are available at the main door of the Gonda building. Inquire at an information desk. Most restrooms are equipped with baby-changing tables. "Family Restrooms" are extra large in order to accommodate strollers. Bottles can be heated at the Patient/Visitor Cafeteria in the Clinic buildings and on most floors of the hospitals. Babysitting services can be arranged through the front desk of most hotels.

## Emergency

In case of emergency, call 911 from any phone.

# Getting Your Bearings

Finding your way around Mayo Clinic can be a daunting proposition, especially on your first day. Since many of the first day's appointments are likely to include a stop at one or more desks on the Subway Level—for example, Desk C (blood draw) in the Hilton Building and possibly at Gonda SL-W (electrocardiography and preoperative evaluation center)—*it is highly recommended that you begin the day by finding the piano in the Gonda Subway Level atrium.* If you began your visit on the main floor

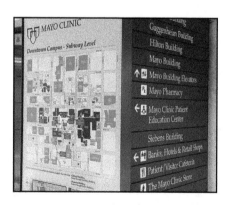

Lobby Level, take the elevators or grand staircase down to the Subway Level. The piano is located directly under the large "Man and Freedom" sculpture at the south end of the Nathan Landow Atrium.

Stand at the piano and face the elevator banks. On the right there are two banks of elevators serving the Gonda Building, Floors SL-10 and Floors 12-19. On the left, there are two sets of elevators serving the Mayo Buildings, Floors SL-10 and Floors 11-19. Occasionally the piano is moved for use in another location, so you may want to use the "Man and Freedom" sculpture as your landmark. The piano is usually located in front of the glass wall near the door to the outside patio.

### Insider Tip

Since Floors 1 through 10 and 12 through 18 of the Mayo Building and the Gonda Building are connected, you may take either the Mayo or the Gonda elevators to these floors and reach your destination.

Approach the elevator bank and you will find a tall three-sided column with signs pointing the directions to various buildings and departments. If you stand directly in front of it, you will notice that to your left is the Mayo Building, Mayo Clinic Pharmacy, and—in the distance—a large sign that reads "Desk C" (in the Hilton Building). If you look to the right, you will see the entrance to the Geffen Auditorium, a large information desk (staffed by General Service employees), the magnificent marble staircase leading up to the admissions desk, the Shops at Gonda just behind the staircase, and—in the distance—Gonda SL-W, the Patient Communication Center, and further down the corridor, the Charlton/Eisenberg Buildings (Rochester Methodist Hospital).

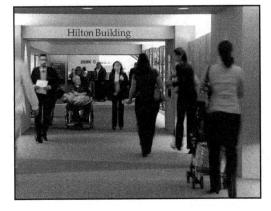

If you turn around 180 degrees and look behind you, you will see a smaller information desk (staffed by volunteers), the entrance to the Patient/Visitor Cafeteria, and a Subway corridor leading to the Siebens Building, Mayo Clinic Store, the Patient Education Center, and—in the distance—straight ahead to the Marriott Subway Level shopping and eating area. Near the Mayo Clinic Store you will find a Subway corridor to the left leading to the Kahler Grand Hotel Subway Level stores.

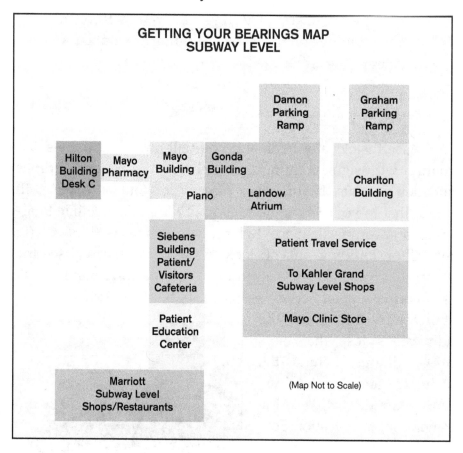

**GETTING YOUR BEARINGS MAP**
**SUBWAY LEVEL**

Damon Parking Ramp

Graham Parking Ramp

Hilton Building Desk C

Mayo Pharmacy

Mayo Building

Gonda Building

Piano

Landow Atrium

Charlton Building

Siebens Building Patient/ Visitors Cafeteria

Patient Travel Service

To Kahler Grand Subway Level Shops

Patient Education Center

Mayo Clinic Store

Marriott Subway Level Shops/Restaurants

(Map Not to Scale)

## Know Your Mayo Clinic Floors

You will not find any directory of medical departments on the Lobby and Subway Levels of the main Clinic buildings. In most medical centers, if you had an appointment with a cardiologist, you would be directed to "Cardiology, fifth floor." Not at Mayo. You will be directed on the Appointment Schedule and Instructions to a specific location, — for example, "Gonda 5 South." Once you get to Gonda 5 South you will find a directory of the Department of Cardiology and a list of the physicians on either side of the reception desk.

The Clinic expects to expand in the years ahead, and some departments may very well move from one floor to another.

As of this writing, the following departments are located in the *Gonda Building*:

### Subway Level
Electrocardiography (SL-W)
Preoperative Evaluation (SL-W)
The Shops at Gonda
Patient Communication Center
Geffen Auditorium
Landow Atrium
The Piano

### Lobby Level
Admissions/Registration
Cancer Education Center

### Second Floor
Audiology, Head and Neck Surgery
Breast Diagnostic Center (2 South)
Interventional Cardiology and Vascular Radiology (2 East)

**Third Floor**
Radiology (3 South)

**Fourth Floor**
Gonda Vascular Center (4 South)
Cardiovascular Health Clinic (4 East)

**Fifth Floor**
Cardiovascular Diseases (5 South)
Nuclear Cardiology (5 East)

**Sixth Floor**
Echocardiography (6 South)

**Seventh Floor**
Urologic Diseases (7 South)
Outpatient Procedure Center (7 East)

**Eighth Floor**
Neurology and Neurological Surgery (8 East and South)

**Ninth Floor**
Colon and Rectal Surgery and Gastrointestinal
Endoscope (9 South)
Digestive Diseases and Cancer Clinics (9 East)

**Tenth Floor**
Cancer Clinic (10 South)
Cancer Treatment Clinic (10 East)

**Twelfth Floor**
Audiology/Vestibular/Balance Lab, ENT

**Fourteenth Floor**
Orthopedics

**Fifteenth Floor**
Orthopedic Surgery

**Sixteenth Floor**
Dermatology

Seventeenth Floor
> General Internal Medicine, Sleep Medicine

Eighteenth Floor
> Pulmonary and Critical Care Medicine

# Mayo Building

Subway Level
> Mayo Clinic Pharmacy
> Judd Auditorium

Lobby Level
> International Center
> Concierge (in International Center)
> Mayo Heritage Hall
> Department of Development
> Office of Patient Experience

Third Floor
> Radiology

Fourth Floor
> Thoracic, Dental Specialties

Fifth Floor
> Executive Health

Sixth Floor
> Infectious Diseases/ Cardiovascular Diseases

Seventh Floor
> Ophthalmology/Optical Store

Eighth Floor
> Neurology

Ninth Floor
> Gastroenterology and Hepatology

**Tenth Floor**
Hematology

**Eleventh Floor**
Psychiatry/Psychology

**Twelfth Floor**
Surgery

**Fourteenth Floor**
Physical Medicine and Rehabilitation/ Podiatry

**Fifteenth Floor**
Rheumatology/Allergic Diseases/Spine

**Sixteenth Floor**
Pediatric Center

**Seventeenth Floor**
General Internal Medicine/Preventive and Occupational
Medicine

**Eighteenth Floor**
Endocrinology

**Nineteenth Floor**
Nephrology and Hypertension

---

**Insider Tip**

When the Gonda Building was opened in 2001, only
ten of the twenty floors were occupied (amazingly,
the building can expand to thirty floors!). Then, floors
12–18 were gradually added. In fact, plans are to build
out the next ten floors beginning in 2021 with additional medical offices and a five-star hotel! Remember:
The location for all your appointments will be clearly
indicated on your Appointment Schedule.

## Signage

You will notice immediately that the signs posted at key intersections of the Clinic campus are invaluable for assisting your wayfinding. The signs are easy to read and follow. The name of the building you are in is at the top of the sign in green; the nearby buildings and destinations are listed below in blue with white letters.

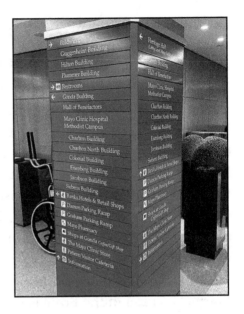

### Insider Tip

The Facilities Operations department fabricates the majority of the signage used at the Mayo Clinic—and they do an excellent job. Randy Staver notes that some patients and visitors depend on the signage to get around, others prefer the maps, and still others prefer to ask for step-by-step directions. All three methods can be used to navigate the many buildings that are part of the Mayo Clinic.

## Information Desks

There are information desks located throughout the Clinic campus indicated on the map by the symbol ? Some of these desks are staffed by General Service employees, others by volunteers. If you come into the campus through the Main Entrance of the Gonda Building on the Lobby Level, you will see a large information desk between the Cancer Education Center and the Admissions and Business Services Desk. If you come in from the Damon Parking Ramp on the Subway Level, a large information desk is located just in front of The Shops at Gonda, directly across from the Geffen Auditorium. If you enter through the Subway from the Kahler corridor, there is an Information Center as you reach the Siebens Building. If you enter through the Marriott corridor, the same Information Center is just past the Patient Education Center, opposite the Mayo Clinic Store. You will encounter another Welcome Desk just past the Patient/Visitor Cafeteria as you enter the Gonda Building atrium on the Subway Level. Other information desks are located on the Subway Level of the Eisenberg Building and on the main floor of Saint Marys Hospital in the Francis Building.

## Concierge Desk

Located just inside the International Visitors Center on the Lobby Level of the Mayo Building, the Concierge Desk opened in November, 2005. Hours are 8:00 a.m. to 5:00 p.m. Monday through Friday, until 6 p.m. by phone—507-538-8438. Ten staff assist patients with accommodations, things to do, recommendations for dining, etc. Although it is located in the International Visitors Center, any patient or visitor can stop by for advice. You can also "chat" with a concierge staff on www.mayoclinic.org.

## Greeters/Volunteers

During the busiest part of the day—from early morning through mid-afternoon—volunteer greeters are positioned at key locations throughout the campus to help you along your way. For example, you will find a blue-coated volunteer standing in front of the Gonda/Mayo elevator banks on the Subway Level, pointing out which elevators to take or how to get to Desk C or Gonda SL-W or any other place.

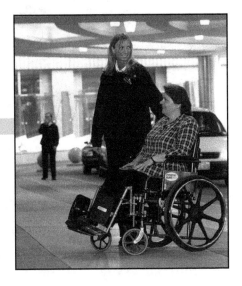

### Insider Tip

The volunteers are well trained to offer directions, advice, and a warm and compassionate welcome. Many of them are longtime residents of Rochester and can give you tips on good places to eat and things to do as well as information about both the Clinic and the city.

## Maps

In addition to the map of Mayo Clinic campus in this volume, every information desk has a variety of maps to guide you around the downtown buildings and the hospitals.

## Admissions and Payment

Unless you have pre-registered or are a returning patient who has received your Appointment Schedule and Instructions in advance of your visit, most patients will need to check in at the Admissions and Business Services Desk on the Lobby Level of the Gonda Building. You will receive your Mayo Clinic "number," the all-important identification for compiling your medical chart, submitting your insurance cards, and/or arranging for payment of your account.

### Insider Tip

The Admissions line starts at 6:30 a.m. before 7:00 a.m. opening. When the first shuttles in the morning arrive at Gonda, there is always a line. If you have received your Appointment Schedule in advance, you can go to your first appointments and circle back to the Admissions/Business desk later in day when it is less busy.

### Insider Tip

When you first register at Mayo Clinic, you are given a "Mayo Medical Record Number—MRN." Amazingly, every single person who has ever been seen at the Clinic has been assigned such a number in consecutive order. Dr. Henry Plummer and Mabel Root, the inventors of the unified medical record, realized that each patient's record would need such a number. For example, my mother, who has been a Mayo patient since she was a little girl some sixty years ago, has a Clinic Number in the 1,000,000 range. I first registered in the Clinic in 1993; my number is in the 3,000,000 range. As of this writing, new patients will get Clinic numbers in the 12,000,000 range!

Patient account representatives can assist you with questions about the costs and payment for your care. You can speak with a cost estimator, someone who can give you a good idea of what your care will cost and other aspects of your stay. (You may get an estimate ahead of your visit by calling Patient Estimating Service, 883-479-5483.)

Ultimately you are responsible for payment of your Clinic and, if you are admitted, hospital accounts. There are additional Admissions and Business Services desks located in the Methodist Hospital, Eisenberg Building, Lobby Level; and Saint Marys Hospital, Mary Brigh Building, Main Floor.

## Insurance Coverage

It pays (literally!) to know your insurance coverage before you arrive at Mayo. Every insurance company has different policies. For example, you may need an authorization from your carrier before you come to Mayo. If your insurance is through a Health Maintenance Organization (HMO), other managed care program, or workers' compensation, prior authorization is usually required. It is your responsibility to obtain these authorizations *before* your appointment. If you need help with HMO or workman's compensation, call the Preappointment Insurance Review Team, 507-284-4366. If you need help with pre-approval of specific procedures, call 507-284-3980 and/or 507-284-0390 for pre-certification.

If you are a Medicare patient, please call 1-800-MEDICARE (1-800-633-4227) to verify the medical coverage Medicare will provide (or go to www.mayoclinic.org for the most up-to-date information on the fast-changing world of healthcare funding). Medicare does not pay for routine preventive physical exams, and there are limits on other medical services. You will be responsible for any "gap" in coverage unless you have supplemental insurance that specifically covers this difference. If you are a non-Minnesota resident, Medicare may not be assigned; therefore, the Medicare checks are mailed to you directly. You are then responsible for forwarding payment for the full amount of the billing to Mayo Clinic.

If you have no insurance, a pre-service deposit may be required.

## International Patients/Visitors

International patients and family members are encouraged to check in at the International Center on the Lobby Level of the Mayo Building upon arrival. Hours are 6:30 a.m. to 6:00 p.m., Monday through Friday (507-284-8884 or fax 507-538-7802).

Concierge services are available at the International Center for both domestic and international patients. Services available include transportation assistance, public notary services, lodging, shopping and entertainment information. The Concierge Services Desk is open Monday through Friday, 8:00 a.m. to 1:00 p.m. and 2:00 p.m. to 5:00 p.m. The International Center also offers Internet, faxing, and printing services for your communication needs. Language interpreters are provided free of charge to patients. Indicate at registration or tell an appointment secretary of your need for an interpreter.

For patients sponsored by an embassy, another governmental entity, or an international organization, Mayo Clinic should receive a written authorization prior to your arrival. The Clinic may ask for payment prior to any unauthorized services, or you may receive a bill.

## Office of Patient Experience

If you have any concerns whatsoever about your Mayo Clinic experience, contact a Patient Relations Representative by visiting the Office of Patient Experience, Mayo Building, Lobby Level, 8:00 a.m. to 5:00 p.m., Monday through Friday, or call 507-284-4988. You may also ask at any reception desk to speak with a Patient Relations Representative who specializes in your specific area of medical care.

## Insider Tip

The Patient Affairs team recommend contacting a Patient Services Representative at any time for assistance with any aspect of your stay at Mayo. They regularly survey these staff members to assess the quality of patient services, often by email after visits. Patients are also invited to fill out comment cards. Patient satisfaction at Mayo is rated unusually high on a consistent basis; nevertheless, the staff is always striving for improvement.

## Getting from Appointment to Appointment

Be prepared to do some walking at the Clinic. Most patient appointments are in the Mayo and Gonda buildings, but some are scheduled within the four-block area stretching from the Eisenberg/Charlton Buildings of the Rochester Methodist Hospital in the north to the Hilton Building in the south. Four blocks may not sound daunting, but there could be a fair amount of crisscrossing between buildings during a typical day, plus walking to get something to eat, to your car, and/or to your hotel.

## Really Big Insider Tip

If you are going from an appointment in the Gonda Building to one in the Mayo Building, there is no need to take the elevator down to the Lobby or Subway. All floors of Gonda and Mayo are connected; simply walk across the corridor linking each floor of the two buildings.

## Insider Tip

If you feel tired for any reason, take advantage of the escort service provided by the Clinic. Even if you don't want to sit in a wheelchair to be transported around, save your strength for the tests and physician appointments.

## Insider Tip

Bring a large purse or satchel to carry the things that will make your day more comfortable. For example, bring a bottle of water, a book, or magazines to read, your Appointment Schedule, and, of course, your copy of *Insider's Guide to Mayo Clinic*. You will inevitably collect many educational brochures and pamphlets. Be sure to have a pen to write your questions and notes.

## Insider Tip

Dress comfortably. Wear low-heeled shoes. Bring a sweater; some of the rooms in the Clinic can be chilly.

# Chapter Five Your
# Appointments

## "Your appointment schedule and instructions"

I F YOU THINK OF YOUR VISIT TO MAYO AS A MEDI-CAL JOURNEY, YOUR APPOINTMENT SCHEDULE AND INSTRUCTIONS is your personalized itinerary. You may receive this schedule in your pre-visit packet, or it may be given to you upon check-in at Admissions at the Clinic.

The Appointment Schedule and Instructions is a comprehensive listing of all your appointments, including the time and place for you to report and precise instructions for how to prepare for tests and consultations. It is typically organized in three sections:

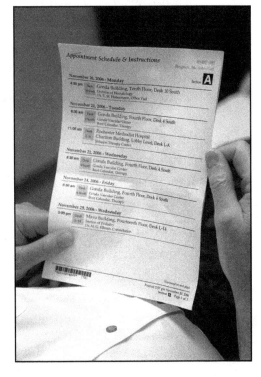

- **Section A:** This is a listing of your day-by-day appointments for tests and consultations. Each page will have your Mayo Clinic Number and name in the upper right-hand corner, the day and date, and a chronological listing of the day's appointments. Within the body of the schedule you will find an exclamation point (!) that alerts you to a specific task you must do to prepare for a test or procedure. For example, nearly every patient at the Clinic must have a fasting blood test, known in Mayo-ese as a Venipuncture Specimen Collection. To prepare for this blood draw you must avoid alcohol for twenty-four hours beforehand and refrain from eating food after 7:00 p.m. the night before the test. Diabetics have different instructions.

Each appointment is listed by time, location, and purpose and/ or name of Consultant.

- **Section B:** This section includes detailed reference information about each diagnostic medical test that will be performed on you. There will be explanations of what the test is, what it is for, what will happen, what you will likely feel, and what to do when the test is completed. This is part of Mayo's commitment to patient education.

- **Section C: Schedule at a Glance.** Your complete Appointment Schedule and Instructions document may run several pages or more. As a convenience for you and anyone accompanying you in the Clinic, this abbreviated Schedule at a Glance lists only the times, locations, and purpose/name of consultant.

If you should lose your Appointment Schedule, do not worry. Simply go to any desk at the Clinic, give the receptionist your Clinic Number and/or name and date of birth, and a new copy will be printed out for you.

**Insider Tip**

Your Appointment Schedule will inevitably change a number of times during your visit. As physicians recommend and schedule additional tests your schedule of appointments will change. A sophisticated computer system keeps track of these changes and how they will impact your preparation for tests and consultations. On the bottom of each page of your Appointment Schedule you will find the time and date it was printed. This enables you to discard earlier versions of the Appointment Schedule.

## Mayo Portal and Patient Online Services Account

With an online account, you can manage your appointments, view your lab results, send and receive messages to your providers, and review your medical record.

The first step to create your online account is to locate your Mayo Clinic number, sometimes referred to as a medical record number. You'll find it in letters from your doctor or on the top of every appointment schedule. Go to www.mayoclinic.org, click on "Log in to Patient Account," and you'll be taken to the Patient Online Services webpage. Click on "Create your account" and you can fill in the information and follow directions to create and activate your account.

To download the Mayo Clinic App, go to your App Store on your phone or computer or visit www.mayoclinic.org/mayo-apps.

If you need help, call 1-877-858-0398 (toll-free) Monday through Friday, 7 a.m. to 7 p.m. Central time.

Mayo has broadened their social media presence with a variety of pages on Facebook, channels on YouTube, and more. If you are looking for advice from fellow patients, Mayo Clinic Connect has many groups by topic organized for tip sharing: connect.mayoclinic.org.

## Who Will You See

With more than 35,000 individuals on staff at Mayo Clinic in Rochester, you may encounter dozens of doctors and allied health professionals during your visit.

The first thing to know is that every single person who works for Mayo wears an official nametag identifying her/his name, a color photo, and area of specialty or job. So if you are ever lost or have a question, stop any person wearing a blue Mayo nametag, and he or she will always be helpful. Why? The Mayo staff is well trained in the art of hospitality and customer service; each person is an "ambassador" for Mayo Clinic.

Mayo has a whole language of terms to describe the people on staff:

- **Consultant**—a physician who is on the Mayo medical staff. Consultants wear business attire when seeing patients in the Clinic. Sometimes referred to as a "Provider."
- **Fellow**—a physician who is training in a specific medical or surgical specialty while at Mayo Clinic.
- **Resident**—a physician, usually a recent medical school graduate, who is participating in a medical training program.
- **Physician Assistant**—a paraprofessional working with Mayo physicians.

- **Allied Health Professional**—a non-physician staff member such as a nurse, laboratory technician, physical therapist, social worker, or patient educator.
- **Clinical Assistant (CA)**—an allied health professional who works with the Consultant physicians to coordinate care and acts as a liaison between physicians and patients.
- **Administrative Assistant to Consultant**—a staff member who assists the physicians with their administrative work.
- **Scheduler**—a staff member who works with the Consultant and Clinical Assistant to schedule appointments within the Clinic.
- **Patient Service Representative**—a staff member at the reception (check-in) desk in a patient care area, an appointment scheduler, or a staff member who provides patients with instructions for specific tests.
- **Patient Relations Coordinator**—a staff member who helps patients when they have questions, concerns, or problems.
- **Patient Account Representative**—a staff member in the Admissions/Business Office who assists patients with financial aspects of their care at Mayo.
- **Auxilian**—a volunteer who works in one of the hospitals.
- **Volunteer**—a non-staff person who helps patients at information desks and as greeters.
- **General Service**—a staff person who works at the Transportation Desk, Information Desk, patient cafeteria, or as an escort.
- **Escort**—a staff member who helps patients requiring assistance traveling to and from their appointments within the Clinic or hospital.

All of these folks are working on your behalf. Impressive indeed!

Once you are at the Clinic, it's helpful to know whom you can ask to assist you with various tasks. Mayo physicians and staff often give patients their business cards or provide you with specific phone numbers you can call for information and help that you may need. The Reception Desk staff checks you in and can assist with some of the scheduling. If all this sounds confusing, do not worry. Everyone at Mayo is extraordinarily sensitive to your need to know what to do and how to do it; it is the hallmark of "the needs of the patient come first."

### Really Big Insider Tip

If you need a certain test, such as an MRI or ultrasound, it is not uncommon for it to be scheduled several days after you begin your visit and are seen by your physician for an initial evaluation. If, however, your physician needs the results of the test sooner—or you urgently need to have the test—s/he can often get you in earlier. For some specialty areas, it doesn't matter whom you ask; the demand far exceeds capacity.

### Insider Tip

In some medical areas you may see a Physician's Assistant or a Nurse Practitioner rather than a Consultant. Know that all of these qualified health professionals are closely supervised by the top Mayo physicians.

## Medical-ese

Some common medical terms you may hear at Mayo:

*MRI*—Magnetic Resonance Imaging—a technique that uses a magnetic field and radio waves to create cross-sectional images of your head and body.

*CAT Scan*—also called CT, computerized tomography scan—is a high-tech X-ray technique that produces images of your internal organs that are more detailed than those produced by conventional X-ray exams.

*CPAP*—Continuous positive airway pressure, a machine that assists with breathing while sleeping.

*IV* (pronounced "eye-vee") "intravenous"—a line inserted into a vein for dispensing medicine.

*HMO*—Health Maintenance Organization—a managed-care insurance plan.

*PPO*—Preferred Provider Organization—a managed-care insurance plan.

*Ultrasound*—also called diagnostic medical sonography or sonography; an imaging method that uses high-frequency sound waves to produce precise images of structures within your body.

*Colonoscopy*—a test to visually examine your entire colon and rectum for abnormalities and colon cancer.

*BP*—blood pressure.

## Tests

Since nearly everyone who enters the Clinic begins the visit with a blood test even before seeing a physician, here is important information about tests at Mayo.

The laboratories of Mayo Clinic conduct millions tests every year! Nearly every patient who comes to the Clinic as an outpatient begins the medical evaluation with two basic tests: blood and urine. You will likely have an appointment time with Desk C in the Hilton Building, Subway Level, for a blood test and asked to deposit a urine sample at one of the many Station S drop-off points in the Clinic.

### General Instructions for Pre-examination Fasting

Since almost everyone begins a visit at Mayo with a fasting blood draw and urinalysis, by following these instructions you may be able to shorten your time at the Clinic. Why? Because if you are not fasting when you arrive at the Clinic on your first morning, you'll have to wait to do these tests a day later.

1. Eat your evening meal 8 hours before your blood test appointment time.
2. Limit amounts of whole milk, cream, oil, gravy, fatty meats, or fried foods during this meal. You may drink as much fluid as you want with this meal.
3. On the morning of the test, do not eat breakfast until after the test is done. You may continue to drink water, diet soda, coffee or tea without cream or sugar until the test is done.
4. Do not take vitamins, iron, medications that contain iron on the day of the test.

5. Continue to take any prescribed medications unless you are told otherwise.

6. Check the instructions for all your tests during the day. You may need to be fasting beyond the blood test, possibly well into the afternoon.

7. If you have diabetes, there will be special pre-procedure instructions on taking insulin and diabetes medication listed in your appointment schedule.

8. If you have any questions about these instructions, ask your doctor. If you are not fasting properly, you will not be able to do the scheduled tests and can extend your stay at the Clinic.

## Station S

When you check in at your first appointment, if your physician requires a urinalysis, you will be given a collection kit—a sterilized cup and instructions for how and when to collect a urine sample. Once you have collected your sample you will need to drop 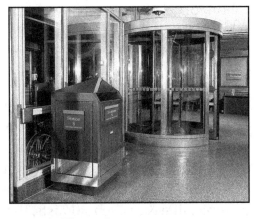 it off at a Station S collection point. These brown carts are strategically located in the labs and at entrances and intersections throughout the Clinic buildings:

1. Gonda Building, Main Entrance, Lobby Level

    (If you are using a shuttle, the Station S is located just inside the building opposite the shuttle drop-off point)

2. Baldwin Patient/Visitor Parking, on both the Lobby/Street Level and the Subway Level

3. Hilton Building, Subway Level, near Desk C or at Desk Desk C-1, Hilton Building. After 5 p.m, samples can be dropped off at Station S, Hilton Building, or, any other Station S on the Mayo campus.

4. Mayo Building, Subway Level (the closest drop-off point if using the Damon or Graham parking ramps)

## Blood Test

My wife Susie insists that Mayo Clinic must use some sort of thin needle for blood tests—they seem so painless and effortless at Mayo compared to tests at other medical facilities. I asked Dr. Hernandez, the chair of Mayo's Division of Clinical Core Laboratory Services, if that was true. It is not. The reason for the ease of testing is twofold: the skill of the hundreds of phlebotomists on staff and the fact that each technician does hundreds of blood draws each and every day.

This is one clear advantage of being seen at a major medical facility that invests in specially trained staff who handle one specific task at the highest level of competence for patient safety. You will find the same excellence in each technician you meet as you go through the battery of tests requested by your physician. For example, like the phlebotomists, the MRI technicians do nothing but MRI screenings all day long.

The Mayo labs are also designed to produce results quickly; no waiting around for days or weeks to get the findings back to the physicians. Depending on the time necessary to process the test, the Consultant staff can count on having access to the test results on the patient's electronic chart in short order.

## Preparing for Tests

You will receive explicit instructions on how to prepare for each test you have at Mayo Clinic. Most of these directions will be included in your Appointment Schedule. Some tests require you to purchase supplies at a pharmacy, to take medications or "tracer" pills, to fast after a certain time the night before a test, etc. Follow these instructions carefully; if you are not properly "prepped" for a test, it will have to be rescheduled, extending your time at the Clinic.

## Taking Tests

Before each exam or procedure, ask at the reception desk how long will it take. Find out how long the family should expect to wait for you. Do they have time to go have lunch and come back?

Once you are in the test itself, ask the health care provider: "What is this for? What should I expect?" Some equipment makes clunky sounds, so don't be surprised; you're already anxious. It is an experience similar to when the landing gear on an airplane deploys—if you don't know the sound, it can be very jarring. Some tests involve flashing lights and strange sounds. Sometimes you are asked to wear a heart or blood pressure monitor for a period of time. Keep asking questions as an active participant in the process.

## Individualized Testing

These descriptions of testing are not meant to cover all tests that could be performed and are general statements about what the author has encountered at Mayo. Each patient's situation is unique, and he/she will be given individualized instructions by the Mayo medical team at the time the appointment is made.

## Checking in at Your Desk

When you arrive at the location of your appointment, you will be greeted by an electronic Check-In kiosk. If you like to use these self-serve machines, go ahead and follow the on-screen instructions. You will check-in earlier than those standing in line. If not, stand in the designated line in front of the reception desk and wait for a receptionist to invite you forward. This is done to protect the privacy of those patients who are sharing information with the staff. Once you are called forward, the receptionist will ask for your Clinic number, your birthdate, or you can hand her/him your Appointment Schedule and Instructions and check you in, usually by swiping the bar code located on the bottom of the schedule (it contains your Clinic Number). You may be asked

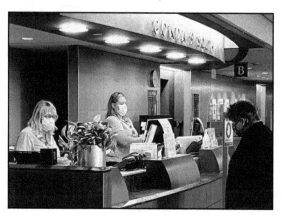

some questions (such as "Are you fasting?") to determine if you are ready for the scheduled test and/or examination. You will then be asked to take a seat in the waiting area until you are called for your appointment.

### Insider Tip

Judy Buckingham, a veteran reception desk staffer, suggests the following, especially for new patients:

1. Read your Appointment Schedule and Instructions carefully before arriving at the Clinic to make sure it all flows well.

2. Pay special attention to the information concerning preparation for tests. If you are scheduled for a fasting test—and you are not fasting—you will lose precious time.

3. Know which building you need to go to for each appointment.

4. Bring a list of questions prepared in advance for the doctor.

5. People are often nervous that they'll miss an appointment, so they won't leave the buildings. Ask the reception desk staff if you have time to go off campus for lunch.

6. Don't be overwhelmed by the amount of information. Collect the booklets and brochures for use later.

7. Understand that one appointment can grow into three or four.

8. Be patient. That's what "patient" means.

## Really Big Insider Tip

You may ask the reception desk staffer to print out a second copy of your Appointment Schedule and Instructions "Schedule at a Glance" to give to your accompanying family member/friend. Due to privacy laws, only you, the patient, can request this. It's very helpful for your family/friend to know this schedule in order to plan ahead for your next moves after each appointment. Or, add your caregiver to your Mayo Portal account for instant access to all your appointments.

# "Checkers"

Every day at Mayo Clinic thousands of patients are going to thousands of appointments. Sometimes patients will miss a previously scheduled appointment for one reason or another: a doctor decides to rearrange the order of tests, a consultation takes longer than expected, someone forgets an appointment. When a patient fails to show up for a scheduled appointment, a slot opens up. Rather than have staff or equipment sit idly by, the Clinic would prefer to treat someone in this open slot. If you are able to have the appointment earlier than scheduled, you may complete your Mayo visit sooner than expected. Just like standby passengers hoping to snag a no-show's empty seat on a flight, the Clinic has devised a system to fit in patients who want to try to be seen earlier than their scheduled appointments. It is called "checkers."

A "checker" is a Mayo Clinic patient who checks at a Reception Desk to ask if it is possible to be seen by a physician or to take a test earlier than scheduled. You must have a scheduled appointment. Each desk keeps close track of how many patients have shown up for their appointments. The desk receptionist will tell you immediately whether checkers are being accepted and your probability of being seen. It is worth trying; you can often save significant time at the Clinic using the checker system. You can also check at the main Admissions desk in the lobby of the Gonda Building, windows 17 and 18.

Here's an example: It's Tuesday morning, and you have a scheduled appointment to have an ultrasound test on Thursday afternoon. If somehow you can get the test done earlier, your chances of completing your visit to the Clinic before the weekend improve. You have no scheduled appointments until Tuesday afternoon; the morning is free. You go to the ultrasound desk (at the same location indicated on your Schedule of Appointments for Thursday) and tell the receptionist that you want to be a checker.

Ask what the chances are of being seen earlier. You'll get one of two responses: 1) "There's a chance" or 2) "I'm sorry; there are no openings." If it's "I'm sorry," don't stay. If there is a chance you can be fit in or you are willing to hang around to see if there is a no-show, you will be invited to sit in the waiting area and wait. Ask when you should check back to find out if you can be seen. Experienced checkers come fasting (since many tests require you to have an empty digestive system) and prepared with reading material. There is no guarantee that you will get in, but if you do, you could save significant time.

Here is the actual instruction card given to Gonda 3 South Ultrasound Standby Patients:

---

We try to accommodate patient appointments as expeditiously as possible. When appointment times are filled several days in advance, you may choose to check for a possible cancellation. If a scheduled patient does not show up for an appointment, that time becomes available. Patients are scheduled into appropriate time slots depending on the area of the body to be scanned and the available time. This means that we cannot honor the "first-come-first-served" rule. **You must have at least four consecutive hours during which you have no other appointments scheduled. If your patient appointment guide instructs you to be fasting for your scheduled appointment, please report fasting when checking for an earlier appointment.**

It is your choice to wait for a possible cancellation. If this does not work out for you, you may keep your scheduled appointment. If you have further questions, the patient service representatives at Gonda 3 South desk will be happy to assist you. We are making every effort to provide the earliest possible appointment.

---

## Insider Tip

Reception desks open at different times, so check in advance. Most desks are open by 8:00 a.m. Checkers are taken at some desks on a first-come, first-served basis, so if you decide to do this, check in early in the morning. By 11:00 a.m. or so, the receptionist will be able to tell you whether you'll get in.

If you don't get in, check in again when the afternoon schedule of appointments begins, usually at 1:00 p.m. or so. You can go have lunch unless the test you are hoping to have requires fasting. Be patient—and pleasant—with the desk people; they will try to get you in as a checker, but it's not up to them. Availability is always dependent on the number of no-shows (if any), the type of test you need, and the schedules of the physicians.

## Really Big Insider Tip

Someone accompanying you may be able to get you on the checker list. Let's say you are waiting at Desk C to have a blood test early on Monday morning, and you have no other appointments until the afternoon. Your scheduled appointment with Cardiology is not until Wednesday afternoon. Send one of your family members or friends to Gonda Desk 5 West to put you on the checker list to see a cardiologist later in the morning.

# Waiting Room Wisdom

Have you have ever been on a water-based amusement park ride with a large sign that says "You Will Get Wet"? At Mayo it would say: "You Will Wait!" During your stay at the Clinic you will undoubtedly spend time waiting for your appointed test or consultation. There are two reasons you will wait:

  i.  Thousands of people come to the Clinic every day;
  ii. The Mayo Model of Care ensures that every patient will be given whatever time she/he needs.

So the best advice is to prepare for the waiting by bringing along something to read or do. The good folks at Mayo have also stocked the waiting rooms with current magazines, Mayo TV patient education channels; loads of medical education brochures; computers for Internet surfing of medical information; Wi-Fi connectivity; and, in some areas designed for children, television sets.

## Making New Friends

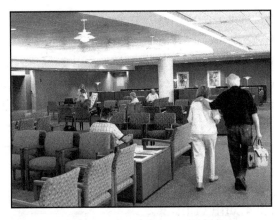

There is a kind of "we're all in the same boat" feeling among those sitting in Mayo Clinic waiting rooms. Inevitably someone will begin to chat with people sitting nearby about the weather, the good places to eat, even the Mayo experience. Some will share war stories of their battles with illness. In the hospital waiting room, especially on a surgical floor, this sharing can be an invaluable way to pass the time while awaiting news. It is difficult to be alone at a time filled with anxiety and concern. Take the opportunity to interact with those around you. These new friends can become an important source of support and strength.

## Meeting Your Physician

It is very important to prepare for your time with Mayo Clinic physicians. You have an extraordinary opportunity to ask questions of some of the most knowledgeable doctors in the world. They expect your questions and are very skilled at explaining the most complicated medical information in language you will understand. The Mayo doctors recommend you compile a list of the most important questions on your mind before you meet with them. In the back of this book you will a find "My Questions for the Doctors" page on which to write your questions. Bring a complete accounting of the medications you are taking; use the form in this guide to compile your list.

Most patients will meet with their primary Mayo Clinic doctor twice: once at the beginning of the visit and once at the end. After the first visit, the doctor will recommend a set of tests to help diagnose your condition. The results of these tests will be sent to your doctor who, based on the findings, may schedule additional tests. Other doctors may wish to see you before the conclusion of your visit to review a specific test result. In virtually all cases, your "exit" visit will present you with a comprehensive diagnosis and a plan of treatment or treatment options to discuss with you.

**Insider Tip**

If you need to return to Mayo for the condition you were diagnosed or treated for, you'll likely see the same primary consultant you started with if he/she is available.

**Insider Tip**

If you want to learn about Mayo doctors, you may read their biographies online at **www.mayoclinic.org**.

1. Click on "Mayo Clinic campus in Minnesota"

2. Click on "Menu"

3. Click on "Find a Doctor"

The first thing you will notice when you enter an examination room at Mayo Clinic is how very different it is from examination rooms in other medical offices. In most such rooms there is an exam table, a variety of scopes, cuffs, and lights, a sink, a desk for the physician, and maybe two chairs. At Mayo Clinic there is a long 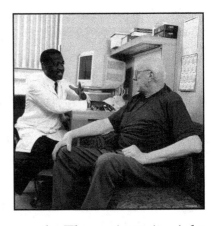 couch with seating for three or four people. The patient sits right next to the doctor's desk, with family members and/or friends sitting with her/him. The physician has a computer on the desk to access the patient electronic medical record. There is a small changing area in one corner of the room with a privacy curtain. In the middle of the room, there is an exam table.

A great deal of thought has gone into the arrangement of the examination room in order to make it as welcoming, comfortable, and functional as possible. In fact, an entire team of experts work in a lab that envisions and models the outpatient experience of tomorrow. Using a methodology of "see, plan, act, refine, communicate," the *SPARC Innovation Program* brings together physicians, business strategists and designers to redefine how health care is delivered at the Mayo Clinic.

The consultation itself will likely begin with a nurse announcing your name and bringing you into the exam room floor. You may be weighed and meaasured, your temperature may be taken, and then you will be brought into one of the many exam rooms. Your blood pressure will be taken, usually up to six times in order to get an average. These details are given to the doctor before she/he comes to see you. The physician will be knocking on the door before entering and introducing herself/himself to you and those with you. S/he will review some of your medical history and inquire about your current concerns. You may or may not receive a physical examination at this point. The Consultant will review your scheduled tests and may suggest additional tests, exams, and/or consultations with other doctors and specialists. The physician's Clinical Assistant will have conferred with the schedulers to set up your revised Appointment Schedule and Instructions. You will be invited to ask any questions, and invariably you will not feel rushed out of the office. Don't be afraid to ask questions or to say "I don't understand; please explain my test results again." Do not hide anything about yourself that is related to your health; for example, if you're struggling with drugs or alcohol, tell your doctor.

Insider Tip

If you don't want to mention something about your health in front of loved ones/companions, wait until you are alone with the doctor. You may always ask to be seen alone on the initial visit and bring family members on subsequent visits.

After this initial meeting with your primary Consultant you will begin or continue your scheduled appointments and tests. These tests will give your physician and other specialists likely to be consulted on your case the information they need to know to make a precise diagnosis of your condition. For example, you may be scheduled for an electrocardiogram, a colonoscopy, an MRI, a chest X ray, or other diagnostic tests. You may see a physician who specializes in the diagnosis and treatment of specific medical conditions and diseases. All of this information will be collected in your electronic medical record. Most importantly, the specialists you see consult and collaborate—this collaboration is the hallmark of the Mayo model of care.

Insider Tip

Mayo Clinic is a veritable Fort Knox of medical data. Mayo has maintained comprehensive records on more than twelve million patients since 1907—arguably the world's largest repository of its kind. Originally on paper, this information is now computerized in an electronic medical record. By knowing your medical history from previous visits your doctor can provide optimal care for your current needs. In addition, data from these records—using numbers, not names, to protect your privacy—are invaluable for researchers who study the causes and treatments of disease. Information from long ago can shed important new light. For example, one of the oldest cases of Lyme disease in America was discovered in a medical record at Mayo Clinic from the early 1900s.

## Clinical Research Trials

As one of the world's great medical research centers, Mayo conducts ongoing research studies of medical treatments in human subjects. Trials to assess the effectiveness of drugs, surgical devices and techniques, and other interventions are always underway at the Clinic. If you are interested in participating in a clinical trial, ask your doctor to consider recommending you to a Mayo Clinic study. Or you may be invited to take part in a study while a patient at Mayo Clinic; the decision to participate is entirely yours and will not affect the medical care you receive.

As a volunteer participant you may get access to treatments not yet available to the general public and experience the satisfaction of knowing that you are making an important contribution to medical research that may benefit others. Because participants generally are randomly assigned to either the active group or the control group, there is no guarantee that you will receive an experimental treatment; you may be assigned to the group that receives a placebo. There are a variety of other conditions if you agree to participate; these will be disclosed to you when you consider joining the clinical trial. If you wish to volunteer, contact the Mayo Clinic Research Volunteer Program, Center for

Translational Science Activities (CTSA), 1-800-664-4542 or 507-255-7128, or e-mail clinicaltrials@mayo.edu, or access the clinical trials website at http://clinicaltrials.mayo.edu, or stop by the Patient Education Center, Siebens Subway Level.

## The Exit Consultation

Throughout your experience, you will have encountered thoroughness at its finest. When you have completed all your tests and examinations, you will meet again with your Mayo doctor or care team, who will review all the findings, make a diagnosis, offer a prognosis, and prescribe medications, offer treatment options, and behavioral changes to address your condition. Mayo wants you to thoroughly understand your condition, have all your questions answered and receive the detailed explanations you need. Dr. Patricia Simmons, a pediatric specialist, reflects on the importance of being prepared for this moment, whatever the news. "Here at Mayo we physicians regard the sharing of results as a critical responsibility. If the news is that treatment is possible, the doctor will set the stage for what is likely to be the impact on your life as the disease is confronted. If the news is not good, the doctor will tell the truth with compassion and empathy. Since Mayo is so thorough about everything, the hope is that the patient and family can accept the diagnosis and prognosis with confidence, stop looking for a different answer, and move forward with their care and their life."

If you can, have a family member or friend with you to be your "second set of ears." If you are told you have a disease, remember it's not just you who has it. Every disease affects the family. If you are told you have diabetes, in truth the *family* has diabetes. Ask about aftercare. How will this disease affect my life? How will surgery recovery proceed? What medicines will I need to take, and what are probable reactions? If you will need to go to the hospital for a procedure or treatment, ask what to expect when you go in and what you can expect after. How long will it take to recover?

For some patients, coming to Mayo is the court of last resort in coping with a serious illness that may be life-threatening. Expectations are very high, and anything less than excellence is unacceptable. But as Julie Lawman points out, even the folks at Mayo are human: "People need to understand we are not gods. But, we see many unusual, severe cases, and if there is a chance to save a life, we will do everything in our power to do so. Many times there is good news; sometimes there is bad news. Whether good or bad, we will be there for you, offering support and comfort."

All of these findings and recommendations will be summarized in a report, a copy of which will be available for you and for sending to your physician(s) back home, if you so choose. If your local doctors have access to the EPIC medical records system, she/he can access your Mayo records online. You may be asked to meet with allied health professionals, social workers, and others who can help you assess and prepare for your treatment and ongoing care at home. You will be invited to stay in touch with your Mayo physician should the need arise. A follow-up visit to Mayo may be suggested within a specified time frame.

## If You Are Hospitalized

Some patients know in advance that they will be admitted to one of the three hospitals in Rochester affiliated with Mayo Clinic. Others arrive at the Clinic for an evaluation, and the physicians determine that immediate hospitalization is required in order to treat the presenting medical condition. In either case, when you arrive at Mayo Clinic Hospital–Saint Marys Campus, Mayo Clinic Hospital–Methodist Campus, or the Mayo Eugenio Litta Children's Hospital, you transition from "outpatient" to "inpatient."

Everything changes when you are admitted to the hospital. You move from your hotel to a hospital room. You no longer move around the Clinic buildings to your appointments; most of the doctors and allied health professionals come to you. Those accompanying you may also move; for example, it is much easier to visit patients in Saint Marys if you lodge across the street rather than staying downtown.

The emotional tone of the visit changes as well. The mixture of anxiety and hope ratchets up a notch. The doctors have decided to offer you treatment that requires the support of a hospital environment and team. This may involve surgery or other treatments such as dialysis. The journey from admission to intervention to follow-up care can create a roller-coaster of emotion.

Your stay in Rochester may become extended far beyond what you anticipated, requiring all sorts of adjustments back home. You may find that additional family members and/or friends will want to come to Rochester, both to visit the patient and to support one another.

The transition from outpatient to inpatient is handled seamlessly by the Mayo staff. You will receive direction from your physician and/or a Clinical Assistant. Once you arrive at the hospital you will be led through the admissions process, be assigned a room, and begin your treatment.

See the chapter on "The Mayo Hospital Experience" for further insider information.

# Chapter Six Dining—
# "Where's a Good Place to Eat?"

W HERE CAN WE EAT?" IS ONE OF THE MOST OFTEN ASKED QUESTIONS AT MAYO CLINIC INFORMATION DESKS. The folks at the desks, the door attendants who meet the shuttles, the receptionists, the nurses, and even the doctors will welcome your question and make suggestions. Since there are thousands of Mayo patients and family members looking for a "good place to eat" every day, a wide variety of options are available.

## Mayo Dining

Mayo Clinic itself offers several dining options on campus:

1. **Patient/Visitor Cafeteria/Skylight Commons.** Located on the Subway Level of the Siebens Building, this cafeteria line offers light fare, fresh fruit, desserts, drinks, a full-service coffee stand serving Starbucks, and take-away sandwiches and snacks. Hours: 7:00 a.m. to 2:00 p.m. Monday through Friday.

2. **The Shops at Gonda.** Located on the Subway Level of the Gonda Building just off the main atrium lobby, the Shops at Gonda offer coffee, drinks, and light snacks. Hours: 7:00 a.m. to 5:00 p.m. Monday through Friday.

3. **Methodist Campus Patient/Visitor Cafeteria.** Located on the Lobby Level of the Eisenberg Building, this cafeteria offers a variety of cold and hot foods, fruit, drinks, desserts, and snacks. Serving breakfast, lunch, dinner. Hours: 7:00 a.m. to 6:30 p.m. seven days a week, including holidays.

4. **Saint Marys Campus Cafeteria.** Located on the main floor of the Francis Building. Hours: 7 a.m. to 7 p.m. seven days a week, including holidays.

5. **Coffee Shop in the Hilton Building.** A coffee shop is available near Desk C offering patients who have been fasting a quick way to break the fast.

6. **Patient/Guest/Staff Breakroom**, Gonda 3. Hours: Monday through Friday, 7:00 a.m. to 2:00 p.m. Convenient for those who have been fasting and have scans on this floor.

## Insider Tip

There are many dining options available to patients and family members located within a few hundred feet of the Mayo complex. For example, savvy insiders know that immediately adjacent to the Siebens Building there are a number of fast-food outlets on the Subway Level of the Marriott Hotel. Stand in front of the Mayo Patient Education Center facing away from the door and look to your right—you'll see The Chocolate Oasis at the end of the hall. Walk toward the store, take a short jog to the right and you will see Salad Works, and further into the Subway past Elle Boutique, you'll find a Dairy Queen, Quizno's Classic Subs, Caribou Coffee, Cinnabon/Auntie Anne's Pretzels, Subway, and Bruegger's Bagels. You can easily reach these eating establishments between appointments.

## Insider Tip

If you are on a restricted diet, in addition to the Patient/Visitor Cafeteria, some of the eating establishments located outside the Clinic itself are prepared to serve patients. For example, at the Kahler Grand Hotel's coffee shop, The Grand Grill, clear consommé and yellow Jell-O (red Jell-O will interfere with many of the tests) are on the menu. Don't be embarrassed to ask; most of the wonderful waiters at these establishments understand what you can and cannot eat.

## Insider Tip

For those who must have (gourmet) coffee, there are several options available both within and just outside the Mayo buildings. The Shops at Gonda and a gourmet coffee stand in the Patient/Visitor Cafeteria, offer a variety of barista-brewed coffee options. Caribou Coffee (in the Marriott Subway) and Starbucks (on the Lobby Level of the Kahler Grand Hotel) are national chains specializing in coffee drinks.

## Dining in the City

Rochester is a fast-growing city with a variety of eating establishments ranging from locally owned restaurants that have served the community for many years to national chains offering everything from fast food to informal dining. In a ten-block area of downtown Rochester there are dozens of places to eat, all within striking distance of the main Clinic buildings. There are many restaurant choices on Broadway, the major thoroughfare that bisects Rochester. The Apache Mall features a food court with a number of fast-food outlets, as well as a major casual dining restaurant in the parking lot.

Consult the information desks and the free local visitor's magazines, such as *Rochester Magazine, Rochester Area Visitor,* and the *Rochester Travel Planner,* published by the Rochester Convention and Visitors Bureau (507-288-4331 or 800-634-8277) for help in making choices. See the list of dining choices in the Appendix, although restaurants notoriously disappear and new ones spring up all the time, so call ahead.

## The Dining Guide

You may find a complete list of Rochester restaurants in Appendix 2 and on the Internet at https://www.experiencerochestermn .com/restaurants/.

### THE BEST OF ROCHESTER

Just as with lodging options, there is no Zagat-type guide to the best restaurants in Rochester. However, the local newspaper, the Post Bulletin's *Rochester Magazine* conducts an annual reader poll and publishes "The Best of Rochester" awards listing all sorts of "best of" restaurants—best Italian, best Chinese, best ice cream, etc. Go to the local paper Post Bulletin's website on this link:

https://www.postbulletin.com/magazines/rochester/rochester -magazine-s-best-restaurants/article_e1d9e12e-46ac-11ea-8cb5 -07ae72241c13.html

Check TripAdvisor and Yelp for reviews and the American Automobile Association Tour Books and Mobil Travel Guides for Minnesota for lists. Visit www.experiencerochestermn.com for a list of restaurants by type of food and location, as well as links to restaurant websites.

> ### Insider Tip
>
> Although Mayo Clinic officially does not endorse any establishment, a favorite activity in waiting rooms and at information desks (especially those staffed by longtime Rochester residents) is to ask for dining recommendations. If the name of the same restaurant keeps popping up, you can be fairly confident that the experience will be good.

> ### Insider Tip
>
> You need not be a registered guest to eat in any of the hotel restaurants in Rochester.

## Eating In

Grubhub and Door Dash are easy ways to access restaurants who deliver using these services. As in most cities, the major pizza chains offer delivery service, as well as several local excellent restaurants.

### Stocking Your Room

A number of the lodging options in Rochester offer rooms with kitchenettes, enabling you to stock a refrigerator and do your own cooking. If you know in advance that your stay at the Clinic or hospital is likely to last more than a week, this can be a less expensive option than eating out every day. InstaCart is a good way to order groceries for delivery from major stores in Rochester, including Costco, Wal-Mart, HyVee, Cub, Aldi and others. If you have a car, consider visiting one of the major grocery stores or super centers in town to buy your food.

### Insider Tip

Ask the hotel to put a refrigerator in your room. You may or may not be charged a small daily/weekly fee. Stock it with your favorite drinks and refrigerated snacks. It can save you a lot of money.

# Chapter Seven Patient Resources

## Communicating with Home

SINCE SO MANY PATIENTS ARRIVE AT ROCHESTER WITH JUST ONE OR TWO FAMILY MEMBERS AND/OR FRIENDS ALONG, the Clinic understands that you will want to share news of progress with those back home.

### Patient Communication Center

Located on the Subway Level of the Gonda Building, a welle-quipped Patient Communication Center offers patients and family members computers with free Internet access and Internet connection for laptop computers.

> **Insider Tip**
>
> In the hospitals, many of the "family rooms" have phones.

> **Insider Tip**
>
> If you have a phone card or an 800 access number for long distance, you can reach an outside line from almost any phone in the Mayo complex.

Insider Tip

In nearly all areas of the Clinic cell phones will work. They can be invaluable communication tools between family members.

## Wireless Internet Access

Free high-speed wireless Internet access is available throughout all Mayo buildings.

## CaringBridge

To help patients and visitors stay in touch with loved ones back home and elsewhere, the Clinic suggests CaringBridge, a free Internet-based non-profit service that enables you to create a personalized Web page to post information, updates, and photos about your stay at Mayo.

In turn, you can receive well-wishes and greetings from family and friends.

Insider Tip

It is much easier—and free—to post news on Caring-Bridge than to make numerous phone calls and send many emails. You will be uplifted by the comments from family and friends. Website: **www.caringbridge.org**

## Chaplain and Religious Services

When you or a loved one is coping with illness, the soft words and good counsel of a Chaplain and/or the spirituality of a religious service can offer comfort at a trying time.

### Chaplains

A staff of chaplains representing different faith traditions serves patients and visitors on the Mayo Clinic campus and in the hospitals, twenty-four hours a day, seven days a week. Patients or family members at the hospital may ask any nurse to page the on-call chaplain at any time or call the Mayo Clinic operator at 507-284-2511. The Chaplain Services offices are located at Methodist, Eisenberg Building, Second Floor, Room 2-130 and at Saint Marys, Joseph Building, Main Floor, Room M-61. To arrange a visit from a chaplain at the downtown campus, call Chaplain Services, 507-266-7275 (dial 6-7275 from a Clinic phone) between 8:00 a.m. and 5:00 p.m. Monday through Friday.

### Religious Services

A listing of religious services offered at the Mayo hospitals may be found in Chapter Ten.

### CHURCHES/SYNAGOGUES/MOSQUES IN ROCHESTER

There are nearly one hundred congregations of all faiths in Rochester. A directory with locations and phone numbers entitled "Rochester Religious Services" is available at the information desks or from Chaplain Services.

## Children at Mayo Clinic

Mayo treats thousands of children and adolescents every year, including several thousand patients hospitalized at Mayo Eugenio Litta Children's Hospital, a hospital-within-a-hospital in Saint Marys. On the pediatric floors of the Clinic buildings, the waiting rooms and treatment areas have been carefully arranged to provide children with a comfortable setting. Television sets, computers, and play areas are child-sized, and the décor is welcoming and soothing. Everything about the Mayo Eugenio Litta Children's Hospital has been designed to take the "scary" out of a hospital stay. A dedicated staff of specially trained physicians, along with a full range of allied health professionals, create a warm and wonderful environment in this 85-bed state-of-the-art facility for children and teenagers. Closed-circuit television programming, art centers, library, and special educational programs and activities complement the health care offered here. On May 12, 2006, conjoined twins Abbigail and Isabelle Carlsen were successfully separated at Mayo Eugenio Litta Children's Hospital, a milestone in the storied history of the Mayo Clinic.

## Charter House

A retirement community for independent living, the Charter House is an affiliate of Mayo Clinic located next to the downtown Clinic campus. Home healthcare, assisted-living programs, and on-site skilled nursing care are also available when needed. It is linked to the Mayo buildings via the Subway/Skyway system. For further information or a tour while in Rochester, call 507-266-8572, www.charterhouse-mayo.org, or stop by at 211 Second Street NW.

## Giving a Gift to Mayo

As a not-for-profit organization, Mayo Clinic depends on the generosity of patients and families to sustain the excellent care provided by its physicians and allied health professionals. Many grateful people contribute gifts of cash, stock, annuities, even real estate through a variety of donation vehicles. Contact the Department of Development, 1-800-297-1185 or 855-852-8129, www.mayoclinic.org/development, or email development@ mayo.edu to receive further information. When at the Clinic, you are welcome to stop by the Development Department; one of their offices is conveniently located on the Lobby Level of the Mayo Building, just across from Mayo Heritage Hall. (There are additional Development offices throughout the complex; just ask and you will be directed to the nearest one.)

If you are admitted to Saint Marys, consider a gift to The Poverello Foundation, which provides financial support to those patients who cannot pay for medical and surgical care. The foundation is named after Saint Francis of Assisi (b. 1182), who was known in Italian as Il Poverello, or "the little poor man," in recognition of his humility and dedication to charity. Call The Poverello Foundation, 855-852-8129.

## Advance Directives

You have the right to accept or refuse medical care. However, if you can no longer think and speak for yourself, you can empower your nearest relative **or anyone you select who is 18 years old or older** to make health care decisions for you. You may also want to put in writing what you want done—or not done—in case you cannot express your wishes. **Talking with** loved ones, friends, and others close to you helps determine your preferences concerning end-of-life treatments. Make certain that those preferences will be respected even if you lose the ability to participate in your health care decisions. Prepare a document that specifies these decisions.

These documents are called "advance directives."

- **A Living Will** is a type of advance directive in which an individual documents his/her wishes about medical treatment should he/she be at the end of life and unable to communicate. The purpose of the Living Will is to guide the family members and doctors in deciding how aggressively to use medical treatments to delay death.

- **Durable Power of Attorney for Health Care**. This document authorizes another person to make **health care** decisions for you even though you are not terminally ill.

- **Mental Health Directives**. This document provides specific direction or designates another to make decisions about the use of intrusive medical treatment for those in treatment for a mental disorder.

You will be asked whether you have prepared any of these advance directives. If you have not, the medical decisions will be left to the discretion of your physician(s) in consultation with family. Many patients prefer to have their wishes known in advance in order to guide health professionals and family members. A copy of any advance directive should be entered into your medical record at Mayo Clinic. For assistance with preparing these documents, consult your attorney or clergy person and/or contact Mayo Medical Social Services, 507-284-2131, and a social worker will discuss your options with you. A Mayo employee is not authorized to write your advance directive for you, nor can an employee sign as a witness. If you wish to prepare an advance directive while at the Clinic, completed documents can be notarized at the Admissions and/or business offices at the hospitals or on the Lobby Level of the Gonda Building.

## Comments

As you might imagine, a medical center devoted to research and to the principle that "the needs of the patient come first" will do all it can to solicit your comments and feedback about the quality of care during your Mayo experience. "We value your comment" cards are found everywhere at the Clinic and in the hospitals. You may be sent a post-visit survey. You may even get a phone call asking you to participate in a survey. These comments are carefully reviewed in the never-ending effort to improve the quality of care at Mayo.

## Tipping

Official policy prohibits Mayo employees from accepting gratuities.

## Mail

Mail should be sent to your place of lodging. Cards, flowers, and other gifts may be delivered to patients in Saint Marys and Methodist hospitals.

## Flowers

As you might imagine, several major florists in Rochester do sizeable business.

Renning's Flowers   507-289-1818

Carousel Floral Gifts and Gardens   507-288-7800

Flowers By Jerry   507-282-2771

Sargent's Floral   507-281-2496

## Coat Room

You may leave your coat at the main Information Desk on the Subway or Lobby Level of the Gonda Building.

## Lost and Found

Check for lost items at the Information Desk on the Subway Level of the Gonda Building.

## Chapter Eight
# Shopping

YOU MAY NOT THINK THAT SHOPPING WOULD BE AN ACTIVITY WHEN AT A MAJOR MEDICAL CENTER, but you and your family members may find yourself with time and often a need to purchase all types of goods. Luckily, the shopping options in Rochester are good, beginning with the stores of the Mayo Clinic.

## The Mayo Stores

Within Mayo, a number of shops serve the needs of patients and visitors.

### Mayo Clinic Downtown Campus

The Shops at Gonda
507-266-3320
Located just behind the main information desk on the Subway Level of the Gonda Building in the Landow Atrium, the Shops at Gonda offer Mayo logo merchandise, newspapers and magazines, snacks, candy, sandwiches, soup, drinks and coffee.
Hours are 7:00 a.m. to 5:00 p.m. Monday through Friday.

## Mayo Clinic Store
507-284-9669 or 888-303-9354 (toll free)
This is the main outlet for health-related books and medical supplies at the Clinic. The downtown campus store is located on the Subway Level of the Siebens Building. Hours are 8:00 a.m. to 5:00 p.m. Monday through Friday. There is also a Mayo Clinic Store (as well as gift shop) at Saint Marys (see details below).

## Mayo Hearing
507-284-2903 or 800-247-1807
This store offers aids and other devices to assist with hearing. Located on Gonda 12.
Hours: 8 a.m. to 5 p.m. Monday through Friday.
Another location is at Kahler Grand Hotel, Subway level, Monday–Friday, 8 a.m. to 4:30 pm. By appointment only.

## Mayo Clinic Optical
507-284-3535; Appointment Line: 507-284-2744
Wide selection of prescription and non-prescription eye care products. On the seventh floor of the Mayo Building.
Hours: 7:30 a.m. to 5:30 p.m. Monday through Friday.

## Mayo Clinic Store Sleep Apnea Supplies
507-284-9669 or 888-303-9354 (toll free)
Consultations and fitting of C-PAP and other devices to assist with sleep disorders. Located on the 17th Floor of the Gonda Building.
Hours: 8:00 a.m. to 5:00 p.m. Monday through Friday.

**Mayo Clinic Pharmacy**
800-445-6326
Your physician may prescribe take-home medications.
You may fill the prescriptions at Mayo Clinic Pharmacy,
at the several independent pharmacies in Rochester, or at
your pharmacy back home. Mayo Clinic Pharmacy accepts
all forms of payment. Be sure to have all your current
insurance and drug benefit cards with you. Medicines can
be shipped throughout the world.

Mayo operates six pharmacies located throughout
Rochester:

**Downtown Campus:**
 Mayo Building, Subway Level (just past the elevators)
 Hours: 7:30 a.m. to 6:00 p.m. Monday through Friday
    Closed on Saturday, Sunday, and holidays

**Baldwin Building, First Floor**
 Hours: Monday–Thursday 8:00 a.m. to 7:00 p.m.
    Friday 8:00 a.m. to 5:00 p.m.
    Saturday 8:00 a.m. to noon.
    Closed on Sunday and holidays

**Mayo Clinic Hospital Methodist Campus**
 Eisenberg Building, Lobby Level
 Hours: Monday–Thursday, 8:00 a.m. to 7:00 p.m.
    Friday, 8:00 a.m. to 4:30 p.m.
    Saturday, 9:00 a.m. to 12:30 p.m.
    Sunday, 1:00 p.m. to 4:00 p.m.

**Mayo Clinic Hospital, Saint Marys Campus**
 Mary Brigh Building, Main Floor
 24 hours a day, all year.

**Mayo Family Clinic Northeast, Main Floor**
3041 Stonehedge Drive NE
Hours: Monday and Wednesday, 8:00 a.m. to 12:30 p.m.
and 1 p.m. to 7 p.m.
Tuesday, Thursday, and Friday, 8:00 a.m. to
12:30 p.m. and 1 p.m. to 5 p.m.

**Mayo Family Clinic Northwest, Main Floor**
41st Street Professional Building 4111 Hwy 52 North
Hours: Monday, Wednesday, Friday
8:00 a.m. to 12:30 p.m. and 1 p.m. to 5 p.m.
Tuesday and Thursday, 8:00 a.m. to 12:30 p.m.
and 1 p.m. to 7 p.m.

**Mayo Clinic Pharmacy by phone**
Hours: Monday–Friday, 7:30 a.m to 6 p.m.,
Saturday, 8 a.m. to 12 noon. 507-284-4041 or
800-445-6326 (toll-free)

## Insider Tip

All of Mayo Clinic Pharmacy locations are well staffed and fill prescriptions efficiently and relatively quickly. You may experience a shorter wait time if you fill your prescriptions early in the morning. The Mayo Building is the busiest of the outlets. It is difficult to predict wait times at the other locations, but you can call ahead to see if your prescriptions are ready for pickup.

## Personal Care

Mayo Clinic Store–Mastectomy and Compression Products offers postmastectomy supplies. Located on the Kahler Plaza, Subway level, Monday–Friday, 8 a.m. to 5 p.m. 507-284-9669 or 888-303-9354 (toll-free).

### Nicotine Dependence Center
Center for Tobacco-Free Living
Gonda Building, 18th floor, by patient elevators.
507-266-1930

### Immunization Clinic
Mayo Building, 17th floor
Monday-Friday from 8:00 a.m. to 4 p.m.
507-284-3577
Provides registered patients and visitors age 16 and up to update immunizations while at the Clinic.

## DOWNTOWN SHOPPING AND SERVICES

With more than three million visitors per year in addition to the local population, Rochester has a vibrant retail community. Many shops surrounding the downtown Mayo campus are particularly geared to serve the needs of Mayo patients and their families. You will find clothing stores, gifts, toys, galleries, jewelers, opticians, flowers, beauty shops and day spa, luggage, books, baby and kids' stores, pharmacies, and card shops. Major shopping areas connected to the Mayo buildings through the Subway and Skyway include the Kahler/Marriot Complex (60 stores), the Galleria at University Square (507-281-1364; 50 stores and food court), and stores along the streets downtown. Most downtown merchants offer validation for city-owned parking ramps.

## BEAUTY SHOP/BARBER SHOP/DAY SPA

The closest beauty salon, Total Image, is located in the Kahler Grand Hotel Subway, offering eight stations of stylists, massages and beauty products. Healing Touch is another popular spot, located at the Galleria at University Square and the Hilton Rochester.

## OTHER SHOPPING AREAS

Apache Mall (507-280-7291), located at the intersection of highways 14 and 52, features many stores, including JC Penney, H & M, and Macy's, along with a food court.

### Insider Tip

A shuttle service from the main entrance of the Gonda Building will take you to the Apache Mall.

**Broadway Commons**
25 Street SE
Kohl's, DSW Shoes, Famous Footwear, Michael's

**Crossroads Shopping Center**
1201 Broadway Avenue S    507-288-2907
21 stores—Pier 1 Imports, OfficeMax, Snyder Drug

**Maplewood Shopping Center**
Highway 52 North
Best Buy

**Marketplace Center**
41st Street NW and Highway 52
Target

**Miracle Mile Shopping Center**
115 16th Avenue NW    507-288-2455
35 specialty stores

**TJ Maxx and HomeGoods**
1300 Salem Road SW 15 stores

**Walmart Super Center**
Two locations;
25 25th Street SE is closest to Downtown
3400 55th Street NW    507-280-7733

**Costco Warehouse**
2020 Commerce Drive NW    507-286-1860

### Insider Tip

The local Walmart, located on Highway 63, will send a shuttle to pick you up for shopping. Call 507-292-0909.

### Insider Tip

There is no state sales tax on clothing in Minnesota except on fur and leather. There is no tax on food in markets. There is tax on food in restaurants.

# Chapter Nine Things to Do in Rochester and Environs

ROCHESTER IS A LOVELY COMMUNITY OF 110,00 SOULS, THE LARGEST CITY IN OLMSTED COUNTY IN SOUTHEASTERN MINNESOTA. In addition to the Mayo Clinic, Rochester is the home to IBM and a variety of local businesses. The city has embarked on a huge $5.6 billion project called "Destination Medical Center (DMC, dmc.mn) to grow the community further into a premier global destination over the next twenty years.

You will find your days filled with appointments, tests, and a fair amount of waiting. But once the Clinic quiets down for the evening, or if you find yourself in Rochester over the weekend, there are opportunities for entertainment, shopping, and sight-seeing in the area.

## Mayo Clinic Itself

The story of Mayo Clinic is beautifully presented in several ways worthy of your time in Rochester.

### MAYO CLINIC TOUR

A wonderful way to acclimate yourself to your surroundings is to take the Mayo Clinic tour, offered Monday through Friday at

10:00 a.m., beginning in Judd Auditorium, located on the Sub-way Level of the Mayo Building, near the elevators for floors 1 through 10. A 15-minute film introduces you to the Mayo brothers, their approach to medicine, and the development of Mayo Clinic into a world-renowned facility for medical care. You are then escorted on a one-hour walking tour of the campus. Well worth doing on your first day at the Clinic, if your schedule of appointments allows.

## Mayo Clinic Historical Suite and The Plummer Building

The Plummer Building is an architectural gem, built in the 1920's to incorporate many of the features designed to enhance patient care and physician collaboration pioneered by the Mayo brothers, Dr. Will and Dr. Charlie, and their partner, Dr. Henry Plummer. On the third floor, you will find a fascinating museum of artifacts and historical documents presented in the original offices of the Mayo brothers. The Mayo Historical Suite, located on Plummer 3, is open for self-guided tours on weekdays from 8:00 a.m. to 5:00 p.m.

## The Rochester Carillon

On the top of the Plummer Building, a musical instrument known as a carillon (pronounced *care-uh-lawn*)—consisting of fifty-six bells—is regularly played for the enjoyment of those visiting the Clinic and Rochester inhabitants. Concerts are performed every Monday evening at 7:00 p.m. and at noon every Wednesday and Friday, as well as on Memorial Day, the Fourth of July, Christmas Eve, and other special occasions. If you would like to climb the tower (it is good exercise!) and view the carillon, call 507-284-8294 or 507-269-5193.

Insider Tip

In addition to enjoying carillon music throughout the day, listen for the bells at 9:00 p.m., when they are programmed to play a hymn that symbolically closes activities at Mayo Clinic. The tune is by St. Clement; the text is "The Day Thou Gavest, Lord, Is Ended."

## Mayo Clinic Heritage Hall

A delightful and informative presentation of Mayo historical facts, interactive exhibits—including a steamboat replica!—and displays honoring the philanthropic supporters of the Mayo Clinic mission is located in the Mathews Grand Lobby, street level of the Mayo Building. Open Monday through Friday, 8:00 a.m. to 5:00 p.m. Don't miss the "Hold the Mayo!" cartoons!

## "My Brother and I" Mural

Key moments in the lives of the Dr. Charlie and Dr. Will Mayo are presented in two long photographic murals on either side of the Subway corridor that links the Gonda Building with the Damon Parking Ramp.

## ART AND ARCHITECTURE TOURS

The Mayo brothers believed in the importance of art and architecture in creating a peaceful environment for healing. Throughout Mayo Clinic, wonderful works of art from across time and geography dot the campus. Volunteers offer one-hour tours pointing out the highlights every Monday through Friday at 1:30 p.m., beginning at the Judd Auditorium, located on the Subway Level of the Mayo Building, near the elevators for floors 1 through 10. A self-guided audio art tour also helps patients and visitors see and enjoy the major artworks in the downtown campus art collection. Hand-held audio sets and maps for the tour can be obtained at the information desk at the north end of the Gonda lobby between 9:00 a.m. and 4:00 p.m.

## Chihuly Glass

Dale Chihuly, perhaps the best-known glass artist of this time, created thirteen spectacular chandeliers featuring 1,375 glass pieces in a variety of forms and colors to adorn the new Gonda Building. They are suspended from the ceiling in the west corner of Gonda, best viewed from the Cancer Education Center on the Lobby Level or from the Mayo Nurses Atrium on the Subway Level (in the corridor connecting to the 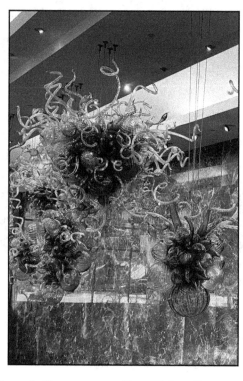 Damon Parking Ramp). The chandeliers are a gift of Mrs. Serena Fleischaker.

## Saint Marys Historical Display and Art

The history of Saint Marys is depicted in a display located on the wall behind the information desk in the Mary Brigh Building, Main Floor Lobby. A display of nursing artifacts and medical equipment, including the first operating table used at Saint Marys built by Dr. Charles Mayo, is open to visitors on the Main Floor of the Francis Building. Stained-glass windows, sculptures, and other works of art can be viewed using a self-guided tour brochure available at the information desks located in the hospital.

## MUSIC AT MAYO

In addition to the Plummer Carillon concerts, music can often be heard throughout the halls of the Mayo campus.

### The Nathan Landow Atrium Piano

Sitting in the magnificent Nathan Landow Atrium with its stunning "wave" of glass (360 feet long and 50 feet high) on the Subway Level of the Gonda Building is a grand piano. It sits there every day, waiting for someone to come along 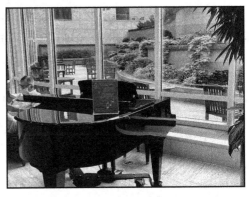 and play it. In fact, the sign on the piano says it all:

> "This piano was a gift to Mayo from a grateful patient. If you feel people would enjoy listening to you, please feel free to play appropriate selections (relaxing and soothing music is preferred). Please do not accept donations, and limit playing time to approximately 30 minutes.

> If listeners wish to make a donation, please leave it at the Volunteers Desk. It will be given to the Poverello Foundation, a fund established to assist patients who are experiencing economic hardships and need financial support for the care they receive at Saint Marys Hospital.

> Thank you."

**NOTE:** You may be requested to interrupt your playing when Mayo Tour Guides bring groups through the atrium. Your compliance with their request is much appreciated."

Every day patients and family members, allied health professionals and visitors who are brave enough and skilled enough to perform in front of a crowd take up the invitation and play. In a matter of moments, dozens of people will stop in their tracks to listen to the music—some for a few minutes, others for as long as the player plays. An audience gathers around the piano itself, while others look on from the "balcony"—the Lobby Level of the Gonda Building. The performer always receives a warm round of applause from the grateful crowd, expressing appreciation for the courage it takes to play and the respite it offers those who walk the corridors carrying the inevitable mixed emotions of this place. The piano was donated by the Kimball family.

### Insider Tip

You never know what can happen when Mayo staffer Jane Belau gets behind the piano. A couple actually met while listening to Jane play, began to date, and eventually got married. They came back for an appointment and told her how they had met!

## Music Is Good Medicine

Music Is Good Medicine is a monthly program sponsored by the Mayo Clinic Rochester Officers and Councilors that provides an opportunity for the voting/consulting staff to share their musical talent with patients and employees. Information regarding each monthly performance may be found at an information desk.

## Harmony for Mayo

A music series sponsored by Mayo Clinic Center for Humanities in Medicine in cooperation with the Choral Arts Ensemble of Rochester, Harmony for Mayo concerts are usually held on Mondays at noon throughout the year on the Mayo campus in different locations. Occasionally performances are held in the evening. Longtime Mayo patients Mr. and Mrs. Tomas Furth are among the benefactors of the series. Concerts are broadcast live on Patient Channel 10 in the hospitals. A schedule can be found in the *Patient and Visitors News* or by asking at any information desk, or go to www.mayoclinic.org/humanities-in-medicine for details on upcoming concerts.

## PATIENT AND FAMILY EDUCATION

Mayo Clinic is a teaching institution, committed to equipping patients and their family members with the information needed to heal from illness and to sustain long-term wellness. Everywhere you go on the campus, you will find easy-to-understand information readily available on virtually every disease and condition known to humankind. In every waiting room on every floor of the Mayo and Gonda Buildings, you will find brochures and pamphlets describing diseases, procedures, and instruction concerning the area of medicine addressed there. There are computers linked to Mayo Clinic websites for searching for information about particular diseases. All of these resources are there for you to take, to read, and to bring home, offering much-appreciated support for the follow-up period of healing.

In addition to the publications distributed free of charge throughout the Clinic, dozens of classes are offered to patients and family members every week on a wide variety of topics: Asthma, Care of Your Back, Fibromyalgia, Healthy Sleep, How to Age

Well, Hypertension, Measuring Blood Pressure, Keeping Your Kidneys Healthy, Stress Management, Preparing for Surgery, and on and on. Even if you are not the patient, take advantage of this incredible opportunity to gain important information about health issues.

---

### Insider Tip

There is a lot of medical information on the Internet, especially at Mayo Clinic health information website **www.mayoclinic.com**. Some non-Mayo Internet sites offer good information; some not so good. Do not self-diagnose. Don't take test results in a vacuum. You need a skilled physician to interpret the test results. Tests can tell you what's happening, but not necessarily why it's happening. That's why you've come to Mayo.

---

## Barbara Woodward Lips Patient Education Center

In addition to the material available on each floor, a phenomenal Patient Education Center is open to all patients, family members and visitors. This medical resource library features brochures, medical displays, videos, books, and journals that can be used to learn about various medical conditions. Much of the material is available free for the taking, although some of the books and journals are for reference only. Moreover, the Patient Education Center offers informative classes every day on many aspects of follow-up treatment, preparing patients and family members for ongoing care at home. Classrooms are set up to explain such procedures as knee replacements. One room has a large photo of an operating room so children are not so scared when they are hospitalized. Another classroom has a kid-level photo of a doctor dressed in three ways: normal dress, in scrubs and a hat, and in scrubs, a hat, and a mask. There are forty-two clinical areas at Mayo. Each group of areas has an assigned Patient Educator and a Consulting Services person to help plan better connectedness between practice and education. In the Patient Education Center itself, an entire staff of educators and social workers provide this excellent resource, open Monday, Tuesday, Wednesday, and Friday, 8:00 a.m. to 5:00 p.m., and Thursday, 9 a.m. to 5 p.m. Closed on holidays.

### Insider Tip

Any patient or family member can make an appointment for a one-on-one consultation or an on-demand class on virtually any health issue. Most people who visit Mayo Clinic, either as a patient or as a family member, have a heightened interest in learning about diseases and treatments. When your understanding of a disease increases, your anxiety decreases. There is even evidence that when a patient knows a fair amount about her/his condition in advance, the time in a hospital decreases!

## The Cancer Education Center

Located in a prominent corner of the Gonda Building Lobby Level, the Cancer Education Center is one of the largest resource centers in the country for patients and family members to access the latest information about cancer prevention, diagnosis, and treatment. In cooperation with the American Cancer Society, cancer educators are on hand to help find information, and offer classes and support groups. Hours are Monday through Friday, 8:00 a.m. to 5:00 p.m. Smaller cancer resource centers are available on Gonda 10 and in the Charlton Building, Desk R. Call 507-266-9288 for more information.

### Insider Tip

For sheer inspiration, read and/or write a testimony in the Patient Journal located in the Cancer Education Center.

## Internet Resources

Mayo Clinic offers five websites:

**MayoClinic.com**
This incredible website offers Mayo information and tools to those seeking information about personal health care.

**MayoClinic.org**
A full listing of services for patients at all Mayo Clinic locations.

**Mayo.edu**
The latest information about Mayo medical research and education programs.

**mayohealthsystem.org**
Offers links to Mayo-affiliated community-based health care services.

**connect.mayoclinic.org**
A community bulletin board for patients and family members to share experiences and seek advice.

## REST

It is not uncommon to hear patients and family members expressing feelings of exhaustion after a day of consultations, tests, walking, and waiting. The Mayo folks know this, and they encourage you to find time in your day to relax and rest. Here are some great places to retreat for peace and quiet:

### Hage Atrium

A skylit area located behind the information center on the Subway Level of the Siebens Building and opposite the Patient Cafeteria, the Hage Atrium is rarely crowded, even on a busy day in the Clinic.

### Nathan Landow Atrium

Since it is located in the center of the Gonda Building opposite the grand staircase to the Lobby Level and the elevators to the Gonda floors, the Nathan Landow Atrium chairs are almost always occupied. Many people enjoy sitting in the outside area, weather permitting.

### Quiet Room

Nearby on the Subway level of the Gonda Building, Room 148, you'll find a quiet room for patients and family members.

### Mayo Center for the Spirit

Opposite the Mayo Pharmacy on the Subway Level of the Mayo Building, you will find the lovely Mayo Center for the Spirit, a non-denominational meditation space. Upon entering, there is a "Prayer Wall" where you can place a personal prayer and several seating areas for your own quiet, introspection time.

## Mayo Building Lobby

Just past the Mayo Building elevators on the Lobby Level you will find some sitting areas surrounded by interesting art pieces.

## Mayo Building Subway Level

Check out the Mayo Peregrine Falcon Cam, a live stream of the falcon nests on the tall buildings of Mayo Clinic. Falcons have been nesting here since 1987!

## Annenberg Plaza

If the weather is nice, a wonderful place to rest outside is the Annenberg Plaza, bordered by the Mayo Building to the west and the Plummer and Siebens buildings to the east. This pedestrian mall offers seating areas.

## Feith Family Statuary Park

Just opposite the Main Entrance to the Gonda Building, you will find a lovely small park featuring statues of the Mayo brothers and benches. It's called Feith Family Statuary Park and was made possible by the generosity of John and Elizabeth Feith to honor the Mayo physicians who have served them so well.

### Insider Tip

If you stay in a downtown hotel near the main Clinic buildings, you will find it much easier to retreat to your own room for a rest between appointments.

## Dan Abraham Healthy Living Center and Mayo Clinic Healthy Living Program

Dan Abraham, a Mayo patient and the force behind Slim-Fast Foods, wanted the employees of the Clinic to take care of their own health. So, he funded the creation of this fabulous facility that features lifestyle classes, fully-equipped state-of-the-art fitness equipment, locker rooms, a five-star Rejuvenate Spa with sauna, whirlpool, and lounge, plus classes and one-on-one personal fitness counseling. Although the center Is mainly used by Mayo employees, patients and caregivers are welcome to call to arrange visits. I especially recommend the beautiful spa which offers massage therapy for a very reasonable fee. The center is connected to the Subway system. 565 First Street SW/6th Floor, 507-293-2933 for lifestyle classes, 507-293-2966 for spa appointments or on www.HealthyLiving.MayoClinic.org

## Rochester

For a city the size of Rochester, there is much to do. Some favorites include:

### Mayowood Mansion

The home of Dr. Charlie Mayo and his family, Mayowood is a popular tourist site in Rochester. Located on a bluff overlooking the Zumbro River, the 48-room "Big House" is modeled after an Italian villa surrounded by beautiful gardens and fountains. Regular tours are offered May through October; a special garden tour is held in June, and Christmas tours are offered during the season. Contact the History Center of Olmsted County, 507-282-9447, or go to www.olmstedhistory.com for dates, times, and cost of tours.

### Rochester Cultural Campus

Located downtown, this complex includes the Mayo Civic Center, Rochester Civic Music, Rochester Civic Theatre, Rochester Public Library, and Rochester Art Center. Each facility offers events. Check the local newspaper, a weekly newsletter called "events x 7" published by the Rochester Convention and Visitors Bureau (available at most information desks and hotels), or go online to www.experiencerochestermn.com.

## Soldiers Field Veterans Memorial
3rd Avenue and 7th Street SW    507-328-2525

A moving memorial to those who served and sacrificed their lives in the armed forces, located in Soldiers Field Park.

## Plummer House of the Arts
1091 Plummer Lane SW    507-328-2525

This was the home of Dr. Henry S. Plummer, the innovative partner of the Mayo brothers. Sitting on eleven acres of formal gardens and landscaped grounds, the 49-room mansion is open to the public year-round. Nominal admission fee.

## Heritage House
225 1st Avenue NW    507-286-9208

See the way of life in a Midwestern family a hundred years ago. Open Tuesday, Thursday, and Sunday, 1:00 p.m. to 3:30 p.m. from the first Sunday in June to the last Sunday in August.

## History Center of Olmsted County
1195 West Circle Drive SW (C.R. 22)    507-282-9447

This museum features exhibits on the history and life of Rochester and the surrounding county. Open year round, Tuesday through Saturday, 9:00 a.m. to 5:00 p.m. From Memorial Day through Labor Day the William Dee Log Cabin pioneer home and the Hadley Valley School House are open to visitors.

## Things to Do with Children

If you have children with you in Rochester, there is plenty to do—even in the winter.

There are inside play areas, parks, the YMCA downtown, movies, bookstores, and shopping.

## Day Trips and Excursions

If you find you have the time, there are a number of popular tourist sites within driving distance of Rochester:

### Amish Tours

A vibrant community of Amish folk live in southeastern Minnesota, about forty-five minutes from downtown Rochester. Several companies offer guided tours, or you can drive yourself:

Amish Tours of Harmony  800-75-AMISH (752-6474);
   507-886-2303
R & M Amish Tours  507-467-2128

### Cabela's
3900 Cabela Drive
Owatonna, MN  507-451-4545

This is the world's largest outfitter of sporting, fishing and hunting equipment, with more than 150,000 square feet of retail space, displays, even a fly fishing stream! Located sixty minutes from Rochester.

## Mall of America

> 60 East Broadway
> Bloomington, MN   612-883-8800

Speaking of shopping, the largest enclosed shopping and entertainment mall in the United States is only ninety minutes from downtown Rochester. More than five hundred specialty stores, plus an indoor amusement park. Daily roundtrip shuttles are offered by Rochester Direct, 507-280-9270.

## SPAM Museum

> 1101 Main Street
> North Austin, MN   800-LUV-SPAM

Yes, they do reveal the ingredients! The SPAM Museum is located next to the Hormel plant, forty-five minutes from Rochester.

## Mississippi River

The great Mississippi is only a forty-five-minute drive east of Rochester. Visit the many colorful towns along the scenic Great River Road.

## Lanesboro and Mantorville

Two charming historical tourist towns nearby.

## Minneapolis/St. Paul

One of the most beautiful metropolitan areas in the country, Minneapolis/St. Paul is dotted with lakes and gorgeous parks and offers shopping, entertainment, professional sports teams, and good eats. Ninety-minute drive from Rochester.

## Additional Services and Entertainment Banking

### Banking

ATM machines are available throughout the downtown campus area. A branch of Associated Banks is located in the Marriott Subway, Wells Fargo is located across the street from the Kahler, and US Bank is adjacent to the Marriott Hotel.

### Smoking and Guns

Smoking is not allowed in any of the Mayo buildings, nor in most locations in Rochester. You may be surprised to see prominent signs prohibiting guns on the Mayo premises, but these are required signs in Minnesota.

### Sports and Recreation

In a town filled with doctors, you would expect to find a couple of good golf courses. Rochester has eight! (A list can be found at www.experiencerochestermn.com.) There are public swimming pools, tennis courts, excellent and extensive biking trails, a skateboard park, waterslides, sledding slopes, ice skating, and bowling lanes. Rochester has amateur and semi-pro football, basketball, baseball, and hockey teams playing regularly scheduled games.

### ENTERTAINMENT

Rochester offers a lively entertainment scene. A variety of musical organizations present live concerts in the Rochester Cultural Center, and touring artists perform at the Mayo Civic Center. There are nightclubs and lounges in the downtown area and throughout the city.

Two movie complexes offer first-run films in state-of-the-art stadium seating auditoriums:

**CMX Chateau Theatres**
971 East Circle Drive NE    507-215-8502

**CineMagic Stadium 12**
2170 Superior Drive NW    507-280-0333

### Insider Tip

Ask your hotel front desk for assistance in transportation to the movie theaters.

Many hotels offer in-room movies on a pay-per-view basis.

### Insider Tip

Some hotels offer discount coupons for shopping and dining in Rochester. Some businesses give AAA discounts upon presentation of your membership card. Many businesses offer senior discounts on purchases.

# Chapter Ten The Mayo Hospital Experience

## The Hospitals

A T SOME POINT DURING YOUR MAYO CLINIC VISIT, A PHYSICIAN MAY ADVISE YOU TO ENTER ONE OF THE THREE MAYO MEDICAL CENTER HOSPITALS—Each is called "Mayo Clinic Hospital" followed by the "Campus" where they are located, although nearly everyone refers to them as "Saint Marys" and "Methodist."

Mayo Clinic Hospital, Saint Marys Campus (507-255-5123), Mayo Clinic Hospital, Methodist Campus (507-266-7890; for patient room information, call 507-266-7067), and the Mayo Eugenio Litta Children's Hospital–located within Saint Marys (507-255-5123)

It's a very busy operation (no pun intended)!

Each hospital provides services in unique specialties.

**Saint Marys** (507-255-5123; patient room information at 507-255-5123), the largest of the three, provides care for most medical areas. It uniquely offers:

- Neurosurgery
- Cardiac treatment, including heart and lung transplant
- Emergency Department

157

- Rehabilitation unit specializing in care of stroke, spinal cord injury, traumatic brain injury patients

- Ventilator Dependence Unit for weaning patients off ventilators

- Eight intensive care units

- Saint Marys also houses a number of research laboratories, including the General Clinical Research Center, which coordinates a wide variety of patient-related research, Gastrointestinal Research Unit, Endocrine Research Unit, and Diabetes Research Unit

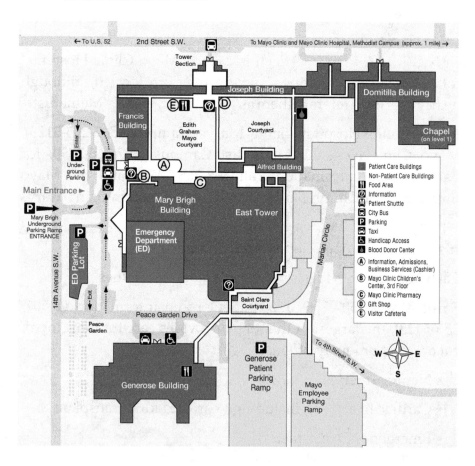

**Mayo Eugenio Litta Children's Hospital**, located within Saint Marys, including a Neonatal Intensive Care Unit, a pediatric Intensive Care Unit, General Pediatric Care Unit, and separate areas for infants and toddlers and preschool, elementary, and adolescent children.

## Psychiatry and Psychology

**The Psychiatry Treatment Center at Saint Marys Hospital.** The Department of Psychiatry and Psychology at Mayo Clinic is one of the largest psychiatric treatment groups in the United States, representing every aspect of psychiatric medicine. The department cares for both adults and children. Many staff members also conduct research and are involved in training new specialists, with forty-seven residents and fellows in training. Most patients are treated on an outpatient basis, but the department conducts several inpatient programs within the Generose Building, the Psychiatry Treatment Center that adjoins Saint Marys.

**Methodist** also offers care for most medical conditions. Special areas include:

- Transplant programs for liver, kidney, pancreas, and bone marrow
- Obstetrics and gynecology, including perinatal center for care of high-risk pregnancies
- Women's Cancer Program
- Intraoperative radiation surgical suite
- Special unit for treating psoriasis and other dermatological problems
- Gonda Vascular Center
- Epilepsy Monitoring Unit

- Nicotine Dependence Center (outpatient)
- Sleep Disorder Center
- Radiation Oncology
- Reproductive Endocrinology and Infertility Clinic
- Colonoscopy Unit
- Vestibular Rehabilitation Unit
- Transfusion Service

There is no Emergency Room at Methodist.

## Pre-admission to the Hospital

If you know in advance that you will be admitted to the hospital, you should arrange for all of your insurance information sent to Mayo before arriving. The best way to avoid lines at the Admissions Desk is to get "pre-certified" for the procedure(s) you expect to have done. If you take care of this ahead of your arrival, your admission to the hospital could take less than five minutes! Mayo will mail a letter to your insurance company to get these authorizations. You, however, may need to update your insurance plan annually; be sure to do this before you arrive in Rochester.

### Insider Tip

The best way to find out if Mayo Clinic is "in-network" is to call your insurance company or plan administrator and ask "What do I need to do in order to get service from Mayo Clinic?" Or "I'd like to go to Mayo Clinic. How can I get pre-certification or pre-authorization?"

They may answer vaguely, because it might depend on the procedures you'll have, but at least you will know if the insurance company is likely to pay.

## Timing Your Hospitalization

As in the outpatient Clinic, summer is the busiest season for admissions to the hospitals. When children are out of school and families have vacation time, many patients plan to have elective surgeries. Winter months are slightly slower. The day before and the day after major holidays are the slowest times in the hospitals.

### Who Should Come with You?

If you can, bring at least one member of your family or a friend to accompany you to the hospital. You may not know immediately if you will have a major surgery. If and when you are scheduled for major surgery, then the rest of the family can come to Rochester to support you and each other.

### The Day of Surgery

If you are having surgery, you may or may not be admitted to the hospital on the night before the operation. In virtually all cases you will be given instructions about (not) eating after a certain time the night before; the doctors want your stomach to be empty when administering anesthesia. You will also be told what to do about your medications and/or insulin. If you are being admitted directly into the hospital, bring all your medications with you in their original containers, along with a list (use the page "My Medication List" in the back of this book).

## What to Bring

Bring any medical support equipment with you—cane, walker, crutches, hearing aids, glasses or contact lenses, dentures and container, support stockings and C-PAP or Bi-PAP machine. You may also want to bring a robe that opens completely down the front, personal toiletries, nonskid slippers, and comfortable clothes to wear upon discharge. You may use a personal computer in the hospital room, but cell phone use is limited in some areas of the hospital. Leave your valuables at home. Bring something to read.

## Admission

Many patients are admitted very early in the morning, sometimes as early as 5:00 a.m. You will be told when and where to report. At Saint Marys, the Admissions Desk is near the Main Entrance on 14th Avenue S.W. on the west side of the hospital. At Methodist, the Admissions Desk is on West Center Street, although the Charlton West drop-off is a bit easier to navigate. After checking in you will be asked to wait until an escort calls your name and accompanies you to a room. Usually you and your family members are taken to a "staging" hospital room, where you are instructed to change into a hospital gown. A patient identification band will be placed on your wrist. You'll be instructed on the use of the hospital bed or recliner and how to view the television in the room. Your nurse will ask you to remove your clothing, jewelry (rings that won't come off can be taped), and any other items on your person, and you will put on a hospital gown, robe, and slippers. Your belongings are placed in a "Patient's Belongings" bag, which will reappear in a *different* room where you will be assigned after surgery. You may be given a pre-op exam by a nurse or allied health professional, and you will likely be asked to give your medical history. You may receive some pre-op instructions, medications, and/or procedures to help you during the surgery.

When the operating team is ready for you, you will be taken to a preoperative waiting room near the surgical suite. The time of your surgery may vary, depending on the progress of other cases. Remember, you will be one of more than two hundred surgeries that day!

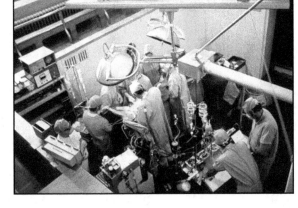

Your family will be allowed to accompany you down the hall to the entrance to the surgical suite where you can have a moment together.

In pre-op your name band will be checked and rechecked, you will be asked for your name and birthday, and further preparations will be made for the procedure. You will have a chance to ask any questions. Someone from the anesthesia team will discuss what to expect before, during, and after you receive anesthesia.

The operating room itself is a brightly lit, very cold, noisy, and busy place. There will be a surgical bed in the middle of the room surrounded by an array of equipment to monitor your condition.

You will be hooked up to these monitoring devices and you will be situated safely on the bed. After the anesthesia is administered, your surgery will begin.

Insider Tip

Prepare the recitation of your medical history before coming to Mayo. You will likely be asked for it a number of times by a number of different health care staff members, particularly if you are hospitalized. This is done primarily for patient safety.

## Tips for Family Members While You Are in Surgery

Your family members will be told which waiting room to wait in while you are in surgery. A "Nurse Communicator" will check in with your family members to keep them informed of progress. Some waiting rooms have electronic boards to follow the status of the procedure. The receptionist will give you a slip with a long number corresponding to your patient's progress on the board. These updates will let you know when the patient goes into the surgical suite, when the operation itself begins, the progress of the surgery, and when the procedure is completed. There are check-out forms at the desk, so if you leave the area, the Nurse Communicator can locate you if needed.

Insider Tip

As you receive news from the Nurse Communicator, you may want to pass along the news to your family and friends back home. There are phones in each waiting room and a phone in the room itself with which to call locally or to use if you have an 800 access number for long distance calls. Depending on where the room is located, your cell phone may or may not receive a signal. Many areas of the hospital offer Wi-Fi wireless Internet connection. Consider creating a CaringBridge page to communicate news.

Don't forget to eat and drink. You could be in for a long day. Ask the Nurse Communicator when you are likely to hear another report so you can judge if it is a good time to grab some food. You may bring food to the waiting area. Take a walk. If the weather is nice, go outside for some fresh air. The Nurse Communicator will likely ask you for a cell phone number or your hotel phone number in case you need to be reached.

As in the outpatient Clinic, the waiting room experience is often a roller-coaster of emotions: hope mixed with anxiety, boredom mixed with moments of high drama, long periods of quiet mixed with excited conversation. You will not be alone. Other family members will be in the area, working the ubiquitous jigsaw puzzles, reading, watching television, even sleeping on a couch. In most surgical waiting rooms a volunteer will appear with a coffee cart, offering coffee, tea, and hot chocolate free of charge. Phones, restrooms, tables, couches, and chairs (some recliners!) facilitate the waiting. Each area features brochures and informational pamphlets describing common procedures and surgeries.

## Insider Tip

Introduce yourself to other people in the waiting room. It helps to share your story, to offer a word of support, encouragement, or comfort when your new friends hear from the Nurse Communicator.

A chaplain will likely visit the waiting room at some point during the day to offer a word of support and, if you wish, a prayer. Each hospital has at least one chapel open during the day for quiet retreat and meditation.

Someone will inform the family when the patient has have been brought to the room and settled in.

## After Surgery

The surgeon and/or other doctor will visit with the family as soon as possible after the conclusion of the surgery. You will be taken to a Post-Anesthesia Care Unit, commonly known as a "recovery room," for a while, usually an hour or two. Nurses will monitor your vital signs and check your surgical site. When you have safely come out of the effects of the anesthesia, you will be transferred to your assigned room.

At this point a new team of allied health professionals on the floor takes over your care. Your nurse will check on you frequently. Your surgeon may visit with you after completing assigned procedures for the day; this may not be until later in the evening. You may have common post-op experiences such as dry and/or sore throat, sleepiness, forgetfulness, nausea, and pain. Nurses will ask you to rate your pain on a scale to help them monitor and regulate your pain medication. You may also be given a self-regulating device to adjust pain medication.

You will also be asked to assist in your own recovery by breathing (using a clever little device known as an "incentive spirometer"), doing circulation exercises in bed, and, eventually, getting out of bed into a chair and walking. You may be surprised how soon after surgery you will be asked to get out of bed, often on the day of surgery. Walking helps your recovery in many ways, but don't do it alone at first.

Your diet may be severely restricted immediately after surgery, and you may experience delayed bowel movements. Eventually you will be able to eat and drink a liquid or soft diet. It's also helpful to know that you can order from the room-service menu at any time.

Oh, and you may be offered a yummy in-bed sponge bath, or perhaps a massage!

### Insider Tip

Each hospital has a massage therapist who visits rooms to offer short massage sessions to patients for a very reasonable fee. Ask your nurse to arrange this wonderful service.

## The Proper Role of Family Members

Generally speaking, family members need to be involved in the ongoing care of the patient. The Mayo staff, as great as they are, will be offering their attention on an intensive but time-limited basis. The family has to learn to be long-term care givers, to monitor systems, to give medications, and to nurse the patient fully back to health.

This is why at Mayo family members are encouraged to be in the room with the patient, even in intensive care. The only exception is if the presence of family interferes with the ability of the staff to give care to the patient. On the other hand, by hearing the reports of the doctors and allied health professionals, family members can become an important part of the team, interpreting the findings to the patient and encouraging compliance with instructions.

Family will be given the phone number of the unit to share with relatives back home. They can call in for reports from the nursing staff, but due to privacy protection, only general information can be given.

## Who's Who in the Hospital

There is a never-ending stream of people who provide for your care in the hospital. Some of them will be physicians you know from being an outpatient; many of them will be new faces.

Some of your doctors are likely to change. Mayo physicians travel with a "posse" of up to five fellows, residents, and interns, along with nurses and other allied health professionals, all of whom work as "teams" on the various floors of the hospitals. These teams make rounds and will introduce themselves to you, as will the nurses, physical therapists, and other allied health professionals in charge of your care. If you are scheduled for surgery, you will usually meet the surgeon and her/his team before the procedure. As in the Clinic, a variety of specialists and technicians will collaborate on your case, consult with one another, and inform you of their plan to restore your health.

Both Saint Marys and Methodist are staffed exclusively by Mayo Clinic physicians. They lead a team of doctors and allied health professionals who provide care and supervise patients in the hospital. This team can be quite large, and you will likely see a constant stream of people during your stay. Here's a helpful "scorecard" of who's who:

**Consultants**—Mayo doctors who are on the staff of the Clinic. All minimally have M.D. degrees, and most have advanced training in their subspecialties of medicine.

**Residents/Fellows**—Physicians (M.D.s) in training for a particular medical or surgery specialty; they assist with exams, tests, diagnoses, surgeries, and other treatments. They are students in the Mayo School of Graduate Medical Education, working under the supervision of a Mayo physician.

**Students**—Undergraduate students in the Mayo Medical School are in a four-year course of study for a medical degree. They assist with taking medical histories and other aspects of medical care under the supervision of a Mayo physician.

**Charge Nurse**—A registered nurse who supervises the nursing team on a floor.

**Registered Nurse (R.N.)**—Health professional with extensive training and experience in health care.

**Patient Care Assistant**—Allied health professional who provides support to the nursing team.

**Physical Therapist**—Specially trained health provider who helps patients regain mobility.

**Respiratory Therapist**—Specialist who offers treatments to help patients with breathing.

**Pharmacist**—Medical team member who formulates and dispenses medications.

**Occupational Therapist**—Specialist who assists patients in preparing to return to work.

**Social Worker**—Medical social service professional offering counseling to patients and family members.

**Chaplain**—Clergy who provides spiritual and emotional support to patients and families.

**Registered Dietitian**—Allied health professional who supervises dietary needs.

**Unit Secretary**—Worker responsible for the receptionist and clerical functions of a patient care unit.

### Insider Tip

Color photographs and names of all allied health professionals are posted on a hallway wall in each patient care unit. This can help you identify those on your caregiving team.

## Nurses at Mayo

Without a doubt, the nursing staff at Mayo Clinic represents the front line of patient care, especially in the hospital setting. Beginning in 1889 with the establishment of Saint Marys Hospital by the Sisters of St. Francis, the history of nursing at Mayo is truly inspiring. Edith Graham, the office nurse and anesthetist for the Mayo brothers, taught nursing basics to the Sisters. (She later married Dr. Charlie!) By 1906 the Saint Marys Hospital Training School for Nursing under the direction of Anna Jamme had become a leading center for nursing education and training. In 1991 the nursing services at Saint Marys and Rochester Methodist combined into the Mayo Department of Nursing. Other departments in the Mayo hospitals employ nurses with other training and background. However they find their way into the Mayo family, the nurses who serve patients at Mayo

Clinic are among the best in the world, the unsung heroes of the medical center.

## Your Room

The hospitals offer private and semi-private patient rooms and an exclusive "Suites at Saint Marys" option for concierge level accommodation, call 507-255-5151 for information. All rooms are equipped with a color television offering Mayo TV, a variety of channels of programming, radio, and music. A number of channels offer patient information and patient education. The hospital bed is adjustable, with controls built into the protective side bars. There is a bed stand with drawers, a dining tray, chair(s) for visitors, and a closet for clothing and belongings.

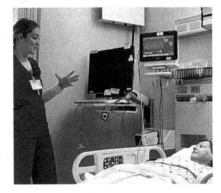

A whiteboard on the wall identifies the room number. Your nurses will write their names on the board so you will know who is caring for you on each shift. You may also want someone to write down your physician's name.

### Insider Tip

Never be afraid to ask for any staff person's name, role, and purpose. Ask staff members to write their names on the whiteboard. Keep a pad of paper and a pen near your bedside to take notes on what the staff tells you, or keep a list of questions you wish to ask the physician and her/his team when they visit.

Most patient rooms have a phone with a direct dial number. You are not charged for local calls or 800 numbers—dial 9 and the local or 9 and the 800 number. Long distance calls may be charged to your home phone number or to a credit card, or you may call collect—dial 9, 0, area code and number. To call international numbers dial 9, 0, 11, country code, city code, and number. MCI access: Dial 9-1-800-950-1111. Sprint access: Dial 9-1-800-877-8000. For assistance with any calls dial "O" for the hospital operator. For those with hearing impairments, a TTY phone can be supplied at no charge—just check with your nurse. Within the hospitals and Clinic you need only dial the last five digits of the extension number.

The hospitals have grown significantly over the years, and it is sometimes challenging to navigate the maze of corridors and buildings. For example, patient rooms in Saint Marys are identified with a room number consisting of a building abbreviation and a four-digit number. The buildings are named after the Sister administrators of the hospital. The building name is a two-letter abbreviation; the first number indicates the floor level, and the remaining numbers identify the area and individual room. Thus Fr5-426 = Francis Building, fifth floor, room 426. Here are the building abbreviations:

| Alfred | Al |
| Domitilla | Do |
| Francis | Fr |
| Generose | Ge |
| Joseph | Jo |
| Mary Brigh | Mb |

The Mayo Eugenio Litta Children's Hospital is located on the second and third floors of the Francis and Mary Brigh Buildings.

## Meals

A room service menu is provided in every room. You may order your meals by calling 507-255-0555 between 7:00 a.m. and 6:30 p.m. You may order your meal for any time you are hungry. If you have special dietary requirements, contact your nutrition assistant or room service. Kosher meals and other special-diet meals are available upon request, depending on your dietary guidelines. Visitors may dine with you by ordering a guest tray (for a fee) by calling room service. If a special occasion occurs while you are in the hospital, a decorated cupcake may be ordered.

## Valuables

You should not keep jewelry, money, or credit cards in your hospital room. The hospital is not responsible for the loss of articles kept in your room. Valuables can be placed in a safety deposit box in the Cashier's Office, Main Lobby, Mary Brigh Building and at Admissions on the lobby level of the Eisenberg Building of the Methodist Campus..

Withdrawals can be made from 5:30 a.m. to 5:00 p.m. Monday through Friday. After 5 p.m. you can ask for help at the main Admissions/Information Desk on the main floor of the Mary Brigh building, just inside the main entrance.

### Electrical Appliances

You may bring a hair dryer, curling iron, electric razor, and personal computer for use in the hospital room.

## VISITOR GUIDELINES

Visitors are welcome at the hospitals, but keep in mind these guidelines:

- General visiting hours are 8:00 a.m. to 8:30 p.m.
- Intensive Care units limit visits; see desk for information.
- Limit the number of visitors to no more than two or three at one time.
- Keep the visits brief.
- Do not sit on patient's bed or in an unoccupied bed in semi-private rooms.
- Children accompanied by an adult may visit during normal visiting hours; children must have authorization from a nurse manager for visits to Intensive Care units.
- Flowers, balloons (non-latex), and cards are welcome in most patient rooms. Restrictions apply in Intensive Care and transplant units.
- Smoking is not permitted in any Mayo Clinic facility.
- Guns are banned on Mayo Clinic property.
- If a family member or friend must stay in the hospital overnight, a Visitor Identification Badge will be issued by the nursing staff.
- Please use public restrooms, not the patient restrooms.
- Do not visit if you have a cold, sore throat, or the flu or are not feeling well.
- Wash your hands or use waterless, alcohol-based cleanser before entering a patient room and again when leaving. Some patients will be in isolation, and visitors will be asked to take additional precautions.

## Parking

Patient/visitor parking is available in the Saint Marys underground parking lot; the entrance is just past the hospital's Mary Brigh Building Main Entrance off 14th Avenue S.W. There is also patient/visitor parking in the Generose Parking Ramp, levels two and three, located off Peace Garden Drive. For patients and visitors going to the Emergency Department, a dedicated surface parking lot is located across the driveway from the entrance. Special needs parking is available from 6:00 a.m. to 9:00 p.m. Monday through Friday at the main hospital entrance in the Mary Brigh Building.

Parking for Methodist is available in the Graham Parking Ramp, entrance off 3rd Avenue NW.

Multi-day parking passes are available from any of the parking attendants. The passes have no expiration date and are valid in all Mayo Clinic parking ramps.

## Additional Patient Services

Mail is delivered once a day. Stamps are available from the mailroom or the Auxiliary Gift Shop. The mailing addresses of the hospitals are:

Patient's Name—Hospital Room Number
Mayo Clinic Hospital–Saint Marys Campus
1216 Second Street SW
Rochester, MN 55902

Mayo Clinic Hospital–Methodist Campus
201 West Center Street
Rochester, Minnesota 55902

Newspapers are available in the gift shop, in newspaper self-service stands near the east patient elevators in the Mary Brigh Building, and in the vending area of the Francis Building, Tower Section, Ground Floor. Fax service is available from 7:00 a.m. to 3:00 p.m. Monday through Friday in the mail room, Domitilla Building, Main Floor, room M-105A. Copy machines are available in the hospital libraries, where you can make copies for a nominal fee. A library cart visits each nursing unit weekly; phone 507-255-5434.

### Insider Tip

If you don't like the art print in your room, you may phone 507-255-5653, and a volunteer will visit your room with a picture cart stocked with alternatives from their collection of hundreds of pictures!

## Hospitality Lounges

Volunteers serve complimentary hot beverages on most weekdays from 9:00 a.m. to 11:00 a.m. on some floors and from 1:30 p.m. to 3:30 p.m. on other floors. Check with the unit desk for the schedule.

### Insider Tip

In the hospitals, a good place to find quiet space is in the Family Consult rooms. If they are not being used by a staff member meeting with a family, these are usually unoccupied.

## Gift Shops

The Saint Marys Auxiliary Gift Shop is located in the Joseph Building, Main Floor, room M-43, 8:30 a.m. to 7:30 p.m. Monday through Friday, 9:30 a.m. to 3:30 p.m. Saturday, and 12:30 p.m. to 3:30 p.m. on Sunday. Phone 507-255-5951.

The Methodist Gift Shop is located in the Eisenberg Building, Lobby Level, open from 9:00 a.m. to 4:30 p.m. Monday through Friday, 9:00 a.m. to 12:30 p.m. on Saturday, and 1:00 p.m. to 4:00 p.m. on Sunday. Phone 507-266-7394.

## Beauty Salon/Barber Shop

The barber shop is located in the Francis Building, Ground Floor, Room G-6, open from 8:00 a.m. to 5:30 p.m. Monday through Friday and 8:00 a.m. to 2:00 p.m. Saturday. The beauty shop is next door in Room G-4, open from 9:00 a.m. to 5:00 p.m. Tuesday through Saturday. Appointments are preferred; call the barber shop at 507-255-5531 and the beauty shop at 507-287-6939. Room service is available upon request.

## Methodist and Saint Marys Patient Libraries

Each hospital features a comprehensive medical resource library with books, journals, magazines, computers, and videos for use (check for hours of operation; typically the libraries are open Monday through Friday from 9:30 a.m. to 4:30 p.m. and on Saturday and Sunday from 1:00 p.m. to 4:30 p.m. Phone 507-255-5434.

Saint Marys Patient and Visitor Library
Francis Building, Seventh Floor

Methodist Library
Eisenberg Building Subway Level, Ei S-59

The patient library provides books, magazines, newspapers, videos, audio books, music, tape players, fax, and copy equipment. The library staff will assist you in finding health information in print or electronic format. The library service is available to patients at no charge.

## Tours

A brochure detailing a self-guided tour of Saint Marys is available at the information desks.

## Patient's Rights

If you have any complaints about service at the hospitals, first contact the nurse manager of your unit. If you are not satisfied, you or your representative is welcome to speak with a Patient Relations representative in the Office of Patient Experience, 507-284-4988, 8:00 a.m. to 5:00 p.m. Monday–Friday. A Patient's Bill of Rights will be given to you upon admission to the hospital with further details.

## Hospital Ethics Consultation

Mayo Clinic is committed to a philosophy of care for the whole person, which includes the physical, spiritual, and emotional needs of the patient, while insuring that the patient is included in decisions about his/her care. Situations may arise when at least two clear moral principles (e.g., autonomy, beneficence, non-maleficence, justice) apply and result in options/decisions that support mutually inconsistent courses of action. That is, some aspects of either course of action will be morally acceptable and morally unacceptable. The Mayo Clinic Ethics Consultation Service will address situations in which an ethical dilemma exists among patients, family members, and medical and/or allied health staff members.

## DINING

Dining at Methodist Patient/Visitor Cafeteria, on the street level of the Eisenberg Building, serves breakfast, lunch, and dinner. The cafeteria is open from 7:00 a.m. to 6:30 p.m. every day, including holidays. Visitors are welcome to have patients join them in the Patient/Visitor Cafeteria. After the cafeteria closes, individuals may wish to use the vending area located on the street level of the Eisenberg Building adjacent to the hospital gift shop in an area known as the Solarium. Hot and cold food and beverages are available at all times.

Vending services including hot beverages, canned soda, and snacks are also available on Floors 6, 8, and 11. A hot beverage machine is located on the 10th Floor.

For a nominal fee guests can also order a tray from room service at 507-255-9999.

### Really Big Insider Tip

There is no written rule preventing visitors from eating in the Employee Cafeteria on the ground level of the Eisenberg Building, especially after the Patient/Visitor Cafeteria closes.

## Dining In/Near Saint Marys

If a Clinic patient is admitted to Saint Marys, there are eating options both within and nearby:

### In Saint Marys

1. Visitor's Cafeteria, located in the Francis Building, Main Floor, offers complete breakfast choices, entrees,

salad bar, snacks, fresh fruit, sandwich bar, and desserts. Hours: Breakfast, 7:00 a.m. to 10:00 a.m. Lunch, 11:00 a.m. to 2:00 p.m. Dinner, 4:45 p.m. to 7:00 p.m.

2. Vending machines are available 24 hours a day on the ground floor of the Francis and Domitilla buildings.

3. Guest trays in patient's room: For a nominal fee, guest trays are available through the nutrition assistant or unit secretary in the Generose and Mary Brigh Buildings. Any other location may order from room service at 507-255-0555.

### Really Big Insider Tip

The Employee Cafeteria on the ground floor of the Mary Brigh Building is open to visitors. This is especially helpful after the Visitors Cafeteria closes for the day.

## In the Neighborhood

Along Second Street there are several well-known restaurants that cater to family members with patients at Saint Marys.

## CHAPELS, MEDITATION SPACES, AND RELIGIOUS SERVICES

There are three chapels at the hospitals, each offering a quiet sacred space open twenty-four hours a day,

Methodist Chapel
Second floor of the Eisenberg Building

Saint Marys Chapel
First floor, Domitilla Building, east end

Saint Francis Chapel
Tower Section, Francis Building, fifth floor

## Insider Tip

There are two lovely areas for quiet meditation on the Saint Marys campus:

- Groves Foundation Meditation Room
  Seventh Floor, Mary Brigh Building
  Open 24 hours

And

- The Saint Francis Peace Garden
  West Side, Generose Building
  Available dawn to dusk — spring, summer, and fall.

## RELIGIOUS SERVICES

The hospitals offer worship services on a regular schedule; communion, anointing of the sick, confession, and pre-Shabbat/holiday visits can be arranged by contacting Chaplain Services at 507-266-7275 between 8 a.m. and 5 p.m. Monday through Friday. Sunday services are broadcast live on Mayo TV, Channel 11.

### Methodist Chapel
Second Floor, Eisenberg Building
Interdenominational Worship—Sunday 9:30 a.m.
Catholic Mass—Sunday through Friday 3:30 p.m.

### Saint Marys Chapel
First floor, Domitilla Building
Interdenominational Worship—Sunday 10:45 a.m.

Catholic Mass—Sunday 8:30 a.m. and Monday through
Saturday 4:30 p.m.

Anointing of the Sick—Wednesday 4:30 p.m.

Sacrament of Reconciliation (Confession)—Saturday 3:30
to 4:15 p.m.

### Sister Helen Hayes Lecture Hall

Second floor, Generose Building

For Generose patients and family members—Sunday
9:45 a.m.

### North Dining Room, Rehabilitation Unit

Third floor, Mary Brigh Building

For rehabilitation patients and family members,
Wednesday at 6:30 p.m.

### Other Faith Traditions

Contact Chaplain Services, 507-266-7275 or 507-255-5780 to be
put in touch with other religious groups offering worship services in your faith.

## SHOPPING NEAR SAINT MARYS HOSPITAL

Directly across from the hospital, a number of businesses cater
to family members with patients in Saint Marys.

# Dismissal from the Hospital

The length of your hospital stay is determined by your physical condition. You will be discharged when the doctors agree
that you can drink and eat without problems, walk with assistance, pass urine, and tolerate any discomfort you still experience. Before you leave, you—and your family members—will

be given complete instructions about medications, diet, exercise, activities, and incision care. If there are issues regarding your follow-up care, Mayo social workers will consult with you and your family about how to ensure you will be safe at home. Your physicians at home will be sent a thorough account of the results of the surgery. You will be given the opportunity to stay in touch with Mayo during your recovery at home.

# Afterword

Mayo Clinic is an extraordinary place. My hope is that the Insider Tips and information in this guide have made your experience at Mayo a bit easier. You may find further tips from Mayo patients at the Mayo Clinic Connect online community—connect.mayoclinic.org.

I wish you good health!

Ron Wolfson

# Addendum Covid-19

I N EARLY 2020, A GLOBAL PANDEMIC CAUSED BY THE NOVEL CORONAVIRUS COVID-19 SIGNIFICANTLY IMPACTED THE MAYO CLINIC in all three campuses. My wife Susie and I were at the Rochester location, arriving on February 10, 2020, to enter the Kidney Transplant Center. Susie received a kidney transplant on February 14 and on February 26, 2020, I donated one of my kidneys on her behalf. Due to complications following Susie's transplant, we remained in Rochester to receive the excellent care of the outstanding medical professionals until late July. During the mandatory lockdowns in March–May, 2020, the Mayo Clinic was a virtual ghost town. This extraordinarily busy medical center stopped all elective surgeries, nearly all appointments, and Rochester itself was eerily empty of cars, with nearly all businesses shutting down. To enable patients the opportunity to receive ongoing care, an enormous effort to provide "virtual appointments" via Zoom and other platforms.The Clinic adopted many procedures to protect patients and caregivers from exposure to the virus. Here is the official notice of precautions:

# Coronavirus Disease 2019 (Covid-19)

## SAFE IN-PERSON AND VIRTUAL CARE

## Appointment availability

Even in this time of uncertainty, Mayo Clinic is a place for hope and healing—and we're delivering the care you need.

Mayo Clinic follows carefully designed, rigorously enforced safety precautions for anyone who needs face-to-face care. We have ample supplies of personal protective equipment (PPE) and full support for COVID-19 testing. Our hospital and intensive care capacity exceeds projected needs for patients with COVID-19.

We're safely treating all patients, both in person and through virtual visits, in adherence with federal and state executive orders and guidance.

We welcome both new and existing patients for virtual and in-person care, including elective surgeries.

**Please contact us to discuss your appointment options:**

Request appointment

## Virtual visits

Video and phone visits can be great options for appointments before, after or in place of face-to-face care. Appointment coordinators will recommend a virtual visit if it best fits your individual needs.

If you are directed toward a virtual visit, you'll want to set up a Patient Online Services account for access:

- On mobile devices: Install and use the Mayo Clinic app (https://www.mayoclinic.org/apps/mayo-clinic)

- On desktops: Access the same services using Patient Online Services (https://onlineservices.mayoclinic.org/content/staticpatient/showpage/patientonline)

## Your safety is our top priority

We've added new precautions to minimize risk of COVID-19 transmission. You can focus on getting the answers you seek, knowing that we're committed to keeping you safe.

When you visit, you'll notice:

- Strict limits to the number of people on campus

- Arizona | Florida | Rochester | MCHS

- Carefully monitored entrance points

- Screening of all patients for symptoms and possible COVID-19 exposure before entering our buildings

- Universal masking required for all patients, visitors and staff

- Waiting areas arranged for social distancing

- Enhanced cleaning of exam rooms and equipment after each patient

- Frequent deep cleaning of other clinic spaces

## TRAVELING TO A MAYO CLINIC LOCATION FOR CARE

Visiting Mayo Clinic safely during the COVID-19 pandemic offers assistance and advice for anyone who needs to travel to one of our campuses or book safe lodging nearby.

We're also working with local businesses that serve patients and caregivers, such as hotels and restaurants. Together, we're creating safe communities for people who need to travel for care.

## WHAT TO EXPECT WHEN YOU'RE HERE

### Please bring your own face mask or cloth covering

Mayo Clinic requires all patients, visitors and staff to wear a face covering or mask while on our campuses to guard against COVID-19 transmission.

### CDC face mask recommendations

Long before you arrive at Mayo Clinic, safety is clear in the details. Here's what you can expect:

- **Appointment request phone call**   When we receive your appointment request, a Mayo Clinic specialist will call you for scheduling. Your specialist will walk you through our COVID-19 symptoms and exposure screening questions. You'll also get specifics on how to prepare for your visit. Guidance for all patients and visitors:
  - Bring a mask to wear when on campus. (We recommend wearing a mask anytime you're away from home.)
  - Follow social distancing guidelines.
  - Leave children under age 13 in the care of someone else at home unless they are receiving care at the clinic.

- ° Arrive 15 minutes early to allow time for COVID-19 screening procedures.

- **Pre-appointment virtual check-in**   The exact method may vary by location, but generally you'll be contacted by a Mayo Clinic staff member one to three days before your appointment. He or she will walk you through a virtual check-in, which may include the following:

  - ° A review of your current medications

  - ° COVID-19 screening questions

  - ° A temperature check (good to have a thermometer on hand)

  - ° A review of clinic guidelines, including use of masks, social distancing and visitor policies

  - ° Information about arrival location and other logistics

- If any concerns are identified, we'll provide you with clear guidance on next steps, including the possibility of rescheduling your appointment.

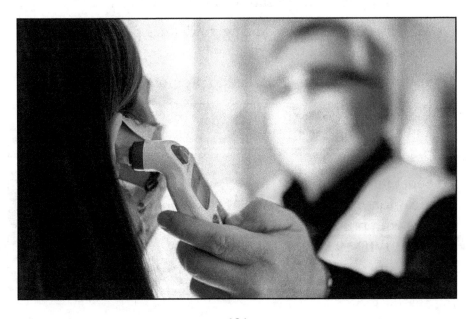

## WHEN YOU ARRIVE

Mayo Clinic staff will welcome you at your designated entrance. They'll guide you through our door screening process, including:

- COVID-19 screening questions

- A temperature check

If your door screening goes smoothly, you'll be reminded of important clinic safety guidelines, including use of masks, social distancing and visitor policies. Then, you can head to the floor for your appointment. If any symptoms or questions come up during your door screening, you'll meet with a nurse right away for additional screening and testing for COVID if needed.

### While you wait

Our staff has taken special precautions to protect you in all waiting areas. You'll see:

- Extra supplies of hand sanitizer available to all

- Masking and social distancing guidelines posted and monitored by staff

- Seating arranged and marked to promote social distancing

- Robust cleaning and sanitizing practices

- Separate waiting areas for visitors with possible COVID-19 exposure

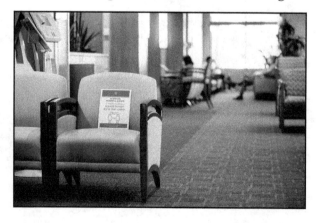

## During your appointment

You'll get the comprehensive, thoughtful evaluation you need from your Mayo Clinic visit. At the same time, you can feel confident in extra steps to protect your well-being:

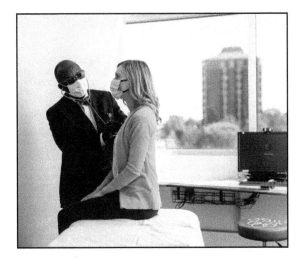

- You and your care team will stay masked

- Consultation and exam rooms are arranged for social distancing

- Frequent and robust handwashing is our practice

- Care is delivered efficiently and effectively while allowing physical distance

- Mayo supports full testing capacity in the event your provider orders additional testing. Some tests or procedures may require COVID-19 testing beforehand to ensure safety. These will be arranged at each specific Mayo Clinic location.

My sincere hope is that by the time you read this guide, the pandemic will have subsided and operations at Mayo Clinic will have returned to "normal." And yet, there will likely be an evolving "new normal," so I highly recommend you check the main patient access point, mayoclinic.org, for updated information prior to your visit to Rochester or the other campuses.

# Appendix 1

## My Medication List

| Name of Medication | Dose and strength (milligrams) | How often do you take the medication? | Why do you take the medication? | How long have you taken the medication? | Date and time of last dose |
|---|---|---|---|---|---|
| | | | | | |
| | | | | | |
| | | | | | |
| | | | | | |
| | | | | | |
| | | | | | |
| | | | | | |

List medications you have adverse reactions to and the type of reaction (hives, difficulty breathing, nausea, etc.)

Name of Medication                    Type of Reaction

_____          _____

_____          _____

_____          _____

List any allergies you have:

_____

_____

_____

_____

## My Medical History

List major illnesses and surgeries, including the year in which they were diagnosed and/or occurred:

| Year | Illness | Surgery |
|------|---------|---------|
|      |         |         |
|      |         |         |
|      |         |         |
|      |         |         |
|      |         |         |
|      |         |         |
|      |         |         |
|      |         |         |
|      |         |         |
|      |         |         |
|      |         |         |
|      |         |         |
|      |         |         |
|      |         |         |
|      |         |         |
|      |         |         |

# My Questions for the Doctors

## Doctor Recommendations/ Prescriptions

# Visit to Rochester Logistics Notes

# Appendix 2

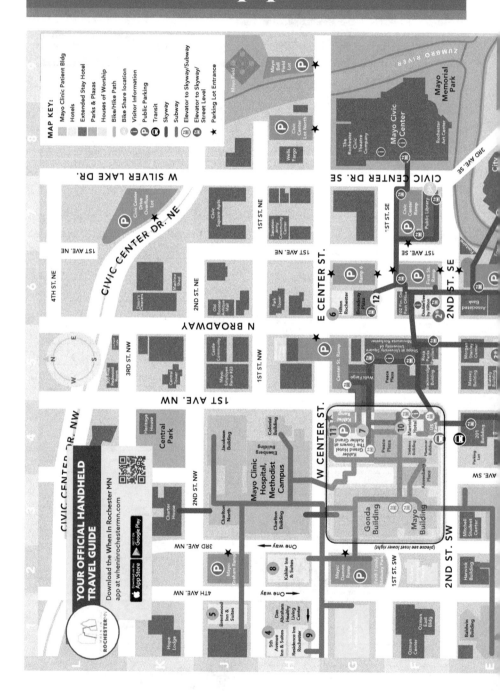

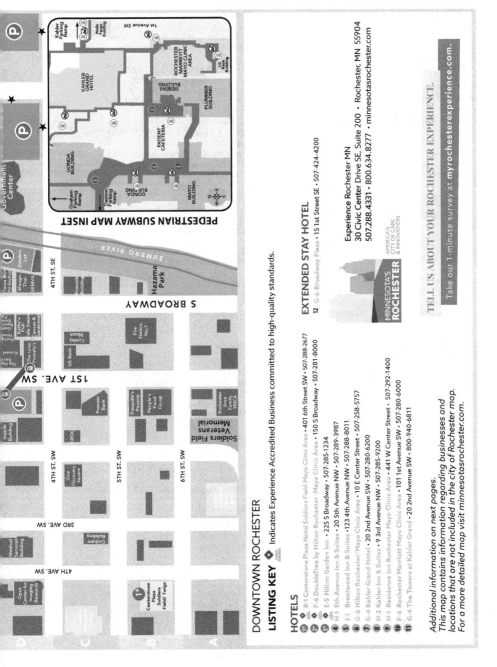

PEDESTRIAN SUBWAY MAP INSET

## DOWNTOWN ROCHESTER

**LISTING KEY** ◆ Indicates Experience Accredited Business committed to high-quality standards.

### HOTELS

1. B-1 Centerstone Plaza Hotel Soldiers Field-Mayo Clinic Area • 401 6th Street SW • 507-288-2677
2. F-6 DoubleTree by Hilton Rochester -Mayo Clinic Area • 150 S Broadway • 507-281-8000
3. E-5 Hilton Garden Inn • 225 S Broadway • 507-285-1234
4. H-1 5th Avenue Inn & Suites • 20 5th Avenue NW • 507-289-3987
5. J-1 Brentwood Inn & Suites •123 4th Avenue NW • 507-288-8011
6. G-6 Hilton Rochester/Mayo Clinic Area • 10 E Center Street • 507-258-5757
7. G-4 Kahler Grand Hotel • 20 2nd Avenue SW • 507-280-6200
8. H-2 Kahler Inn & Suites • 9 3rd Avenue NW • 507-285-9200
9. H-1 Residence Inn Rochester Mayo Clinic Area • 441 W Center Street • 507-292-1400
10. F-4 Rochester Marriott Mayo Clinic Area • 101 1st Avenue SW • 507-280-6000
11. G-4 The Towers at Kahler Grand • 20 2nd Avenue SW • 800-940-6811

### EXTENDED STAY HOTEL

12. G-6 Broadway Plaza • 15 1st Street SE • 507-424-4200

Experience Rochester MN
30 Civic Center Drive SE, Suite 200 • Rochester, MN 55904
507.288.4331 • 800.634.8277 • minnesotasrochester.com

MINNESOTA'S
**ROCHESTER**
AMERICA'S
CITY OF CARE
& INNOVATION

TELL US ABOUT YOUR ROCHESTER EXPERIENCE.
Take our 1-minute survey at **myrochesterexperience.com.**

*Additional information on next pages.*
*This map contains information regarding businesses and*
*locations that are not included in the city of Rochester map.*
*For a more detailed map visit minnesotasrochester.com.*

## RESTAURANTS

### AMERICAN

♦ **Bleu Duck Kitchen** C-5
14 4th Street SW • (507) 258-4663
bleuduckkitchen.com

♦ **Twigs Tavern & Grille** B-1
401 6th Street SW • (507) 288-0206
twigstavernandgrille.com

**300 First** L-5
300 1st Avenue NW • (507) 281-2451 live2dine.
com/300-first

**American Legion Post 92** L-4
315 1st Avenue NW • (507) 282-1322 post92.
org

**Bruegger's Bagels** F-4
155 1st Avenue SW • (507) 424-4777
brueggers.com

**CB3 Burgers + Brew** H-2
9 3rd Avenue NW • (507) 285-9200 kahler.com/
cb3

**Chester's Kitchen & Bar** F-5
111 S Broadway • (507) 424-1211 chesterskb.
com

**City Market** E-5
212 1st Avenue SW • (507) 536-4748 live2dine.
com/city-market

**Daube's Down-Under** F-4
155 1st Avenue SW • (507) 252-8878
daubesbakery.com

**Dooley's Pub** E-4
255 1st Avenue SW • (507) 208-4085
dooleyspubroch.com

**Dunkin' Donuts** G-4
15 1st Avenue SW • (507) 285-2719
dunkindonuts.com

**Freshens** F-4
101 1st Avenue SW • (507) 285-2705 freshens.
com

**Garden Express** F-5
100 1st Avenue SW • (507) 322-0686
gardenexpress.org

**Grand Grill** G-4
20 2nd Avenue SW • (507) 285-2585 kahler.
com/the-grand-grill

**Grand Rounds Brew Pub** D-5
4 3rd Street SW • (507) 292-1628
grandroundsbrewpub.com

**Jimmy John's** H-2
9 3rd Avenue NW • (507) 289-9900
jimmyjohns.com

**Legends Bar-N-Grill** D-6
11 4th Street SE • (507) 424-1896

**Lettuce Unite** F-5
100 1st Avenue SW • (507) 206-4560 lettuce-
unite.com

**Lord Essex The Steakhouse** G-4
20 2nd Avenue SW • (507) 280-6200 kahler.
com/lord-essex-1

**Martini's** G-4
20 2nd Avenue SW • (507) 280-6200 kahler.
com/martinis

**Mattan's Grilled Philly Steak Subs** J-5
101 N Broadway • (507) 288-2188

**Newt's** E-5
216 1/2 1st Avenue SW • (507) 289-0577
live2dine.com/newts

**Newt's Express** F-5
100 1st Avenue SW • (507) 289-0577 live2dine.
com/content/newts-express

**Porch and Cellar** C-8
20 4th Street SE • (507) 322-6551
porchandcellar.com/porch

**Potbelly Sandwich Shop** D-5
318 1st Avenue SW • (507) 424-1661 potbelly.
com

**Quiznos Subs** F-4
101 1st Avenue SW • (507) 292-5725 quiznos.
corn

**Salad Brothers Cafe & Deli** F-5
111 S Broadway • (507) 289-1560

**Subway** F-4
155 1st Avenue SW • (507) 282-7976 subway.
com

**The Half Barrel Bar & Kitchen** D-5
304 1st Avenue SW • (507) 258-6606
halfbarrelbar.com

**The Loop** D-5
318 1st Avenue SW • (507) 226-8644
thelooprochester.com

**The Redwood Room** L-5
300 1st Avenue NW • (507) 281-2978 live2dine.
com/redwood-room

**The Tap House** D-5
10 3rd Street SW • (507) 258-4017
taphousemn.com

### ASIAN

**Chinese Chinh's Express** F-5
100 1st Avenue SW • (507) 258-5350
chinesechinsexpress.com/#!menu

**Mango Thai** D-6
318 S Broadway • (507) 288-2360
mangothaimn.com

**Mango Thai Express** F-5
100 1st Avenue SW • (507) 288-2360
mangothaimn.com

**Wabi Sabi Express** F-5
100 1st Avenue SW • (507) 258-5288

**ZY Teriyaki** F-5
101 1st Avenue SW • (626) 688-4008

### BREWERIES

**Grand Rounds Brew Pub** D-5
4 3rd Street SW • (507) 292-1628
grandroundsbrewpub.com

### COFFEE/SPECIALTY DRINKS

**Almis Coffee Shop** H-5
117 N Broadway • (507) 271-5519

**Bravo Espresso** F-5
111 S Broadway • (507) 281-4076

**Cafe Steam**
D-5 315 S Broadway • (507) 208-4160
F-6 150 S Broadway • steam.coffee

Caribou Coffee
F-4 101 1st Avenue SW • (507) 288-6230
H-2 9 3rd Avenue NW • (507) 280-4375
cariboucoffee.com
Dunkin' Donuts G-4
15 1st Avenue SW • (507) 285-2719
dunkindonuts.com
People's Food Co-op B-4
519 1st Avenue SW • (507) 289-9061 pfc.coop
Starbucks G-4
20 2nd Avenue SW • (507) 280-6200
starbucks.com
Tea Time G-4
20 2nd Avenue SW • (507) 261-9868

## CUBAN

Francisco's Cuban Cafe F-5
101 1st Avenue SW • (507) 258-7722
franciscoscubancafe.com

## DELIVERY/CONVENIENCE

Waiter Express
829 3rd Avenue SE • (507) 288-8883
waiterexpress.net

## DESSERT

Auntie Anne's F-4
101 1st Avenue SW • (507) 281-1233
auntieannes.com
Carroll's Corn G-4
20 2nd Avenue SW • (507) 287-3307
carrollscorn.com
Carroll's Cup G-4
20 2nd Avenue SW • (507) 288-2470
carrollscorn.com/carrolls-cup
Chocolate Oasis F-5
101 1st Avenue SW • (507) 280-6760
Chocolaterie Stam F-5
111 S Broadway • (507) 536-2722
stamchocolate.com
Cinnabon F-4
101 1st Avenue SW • (507) 281-1233 cinnabon.
com
Dairy Queen F-4
101 1st Avenue SW • (507) 282-6633
dairyqueen.com
Daube's Down-Under F-4
155 1st Avenue SW • (507) 252-8878
daubesbakery.com
Dunkin' Donuts G-4
15 1st Avenue SW • (507) 285-2719
dunkindonuts.com
Pasquale's Neighborhood Pizzeria B-4
130 5th Street SW • (507) 424-7800 pnppizza.
com

## FOOD TRUCKS

Jersey Jo's
1st Avenue SW • (507) 258-7555 jerseyjos.com
Murph's at Peace Plaza F-5
1st Avenue SW

Old Abe Coffee Co. E-4
2nd Avenue SW+ 2nd Street SW (651) 410-
4137 oldabecoffee.com
The Back Alley Kitchen D-4
2nd Avenue SW + 3rd Street SW (507) 254-
7249 squareup.com/store/thebackalleykitchen

## GREEK

Nupa Express F-5
100 1st Avenue SW • (507) 206-5044 eatnupa.
com

## INDIAN

Blue Diamond Restaurant F-5
100 1st Avenue SW • (507) 292-9009
bluediamondrestaurant.us

## ITALIAN

Pasquale's Neighborhood Pizzeria B-4
130 5th Street SW • (507) 424-7800 pnppizza.
com
Salute! wine bar & more F-4
101 1st Avenue SW • (507) 285-2766 kahler.
com/salute
Terza Ristorante D-6
30 3rd Street SE • (507) 413-4033 terza3.com
Victoria's Express G-4
7 1st Avenue SW • (507) 280-6232 victoriasmn.
com/express
Victoria's Italian Restaurant and Wine Bar G-4
7 1st Avenue SW • (507) 280-6232 victoriasmn.
com

## MEXICAN

Hefe Rojo E-5
216 1st Avenue SW • (507) 289-1949 live2dine.
com/hefe-rojo

## MIDDLE EASTERN

Kabab Restaurant H-7
125 E Center Street • (507) 288-2181

## PIZZA

BB's Express F-5
111 S Broadway • bbspizzaria.com
Pasquale's Neighborhood Pizzeria B-4
130 5th Street SW • (507) 424-7800 pnppizza.
com
Twisted Barrel Wood Fired Pizza D-4
244 E Soldiers Field Dr SW • (507) 292-9009
twistedbarrelpizza.com

## SEAFOOD

◊ Pescara F-6
150 S Broadway • (507) 280-6900
pescarafresh.com

## NIGHTLIFE

**Twigs Tavern & Grille** B-1
401 6th Street SW • (507) 288-0206
twigstavernandgrille.com

**Chester's Kitchen & Bar** F-5
111 S Broadway • (507) 424-1211 chesterskb.com

**Dooley's Pub** E-4
255 1st Avenue SW • (507) 208-4085
dooleyspubroch.com

**Fusion Lounge** D-6
310 S Broadway • (507) 322-6980
fusionloungerochester.com

**Grand Rounds Brew Pub** D-5
4 3rd Street SW • (507) 292-1628
grandroundsbrewpub.com

**Hefe Rojo** E-5
216 1st Avenue SW • (507) 289-1949 live2dine.com/hefe-rojo

**Kathy's Pub** D-5
307 S Broadway • (507) 252-8355 kathyspub.info

**La Vetta** D-6
30 3rd Street SE • (507) 413-4033 terza3.com/la-vetta

**Legends Bar-N-Grill** D-6
11 4th Street SE • (507) 424-1896

**Martini's** G-4
20 2nd Avenue SW • (507) 280-6200 kahler.com/martinis

**Newt's** E-5
216 1/2 1st Avenue SW • (507) 289-0577
live2dine.com/newts

**The Half Barrel Bar & Kitchen** D-5
304 1st Avenue SW • (507) 258-6606
halfbarrelbar.com

**The Loop** D-5
318 1st Avenue SW • (507) 226-8644
thelooprochester.com

**The Redwood Room** L-5
300 1st Avenue NW • (507) 281-2978 live2dine.com/redwood-room

**The Tap House** D-5
10 3rd Street SW • (507) 258-4017
taphousemn.com

## THINGS TO DO

**Rochester Trolley & Tour Company** F-4
101 1st Avenue SW • (507) 421-0573
rochestermntours.com

**Calvary Episcopal Church** F-2
111 3rd Avenue SW • (507) 282-9429 calvary-rochester.org

**Canvas & Chardonnay** D-5
317 S Broadway • (507) 258-4268
canvasandchardonnay.com

**Harmony for Mayo Program** H-3
200 1st Street SW • (507) 284-5111 mayoclinic.org

**Heritage House Victorian Museum** K-4
225 1st Avenue NW • (507) 286-9208
heritagehousevictorianmuseum.com

**Mayo Civic Center** F-8
30 Civic Center Drive SE • (507) 328-2222
mayociviccenter.com

**Mayo Clinic Tours** G-3
For Mayo Clinic Patients and Guests 200 1st Street SW • (507) 284-5111 mayoclinic.org

**Rochester Bike Share**
G-5 1st Avenue SW (Peace Plaza)
F-7 101 2nd Street St SE (Public Library) E-7 201 4th Street SE (City Hall) rochestermn.gov

**Plummer Building** F-4
113 2nd Street SW • mayoclinic.org

**Riverside Concerts** G-8
201 4th Street SE • (507) 328-2200
riversideconcerts.com

**Rochester Area Family YMCA** A-4
709 1st Avenue SW • (507) 287-2260 rochfamy.org

**Rochester Art Center** G-8
40 Civic Center Drive SE • (507) 282-8629
rochesterartcenter.org

**Rochester Civic Theatre Company** G-8
20 Civic Center Drive SE • (507) 282-8481
rochestercivictheatre.org

**Rochester Honkers Baseball** H-9
307 E Center Street • (507) 289-1170
rochesterhonkers.com

**Rochester Public Library** F-7
101 2nd Street SE • (507) 328-2300
rochesterpubliclibrary.org

**Rochester Royals** H-9
403 E Center Street • (507) 281-0612
rochestermnroyals.com

**Rochester Symphony Orchestra and Chorale** C-6
1530 Greenview Drive SW • (507) 286-8742
rochestersymphony.org

**SEMVA/Southeastern Minnesota Visual Artists Gallery** D-6
320 S Broadway • (507) 281-4920 semva.com

**Soldiers Field Veterans Memorial** A-4
300 7th Street SW • (507) 289-8981
soldiersfieldmemorial.org

**Soldiers Memorial Field Park** A-4
244 Soldiers Field Drive SW • (507) 328-2525
rochestermn.gov

**The Machine Shed** K-6
11 2nd Street NE • (507) 202-6761
machineshedmn.com

**The Rochester Carillon** F-4
200 1st Street SW • (507) 284-8294
mayoclinic.org

**Zerkalov Art Gallery** D-5
319 S Broadway

## GOLF

Soldiers Field Golf Course A-4
224 Soldiers Field Drive SW • (507) 281-6176
rochestermn.gov

## SHOPPING

Shops at University Square F-5
111 S Broadway • (888) 280-6419
shopsatuniversitysquare.com
The Grand Shops/Kahler & Marriott G-4
20 2nd Avenue SW • (507) 280-6200 kahler.
com/areaguide/grand-shops

## GROCERY STORES

International Spices & Grocery H-7
125 E Center Street • (507) 288-8007
People's Food Co-op J-5
519 1st Avenue SW • (507) 289-9061 pfc.coop

## PHARMACY + DRUG

GuidePoint Pharmacy K-6
202 N Broadway • (507) 288-6463
guidepointpharmacy.com
Mayo Clinic Pharmacies
E-1 Baldwin Bldg - 221 4th Avenue SW (507)
284-8880
F-3 Mayo Bldg - 200 1st Street SW (507) 284-
2021
H-4 Eisenberg Bldg - 201 W Center Street
(507) 266-7416
www.mayoclinic.org
Weber & Judd Pharmacies F-4
101 1st Avenue SW • (507) 289-0716
weberjudd.com

## SPAS + SALONS

Blu H2O Salon F-6
150 S Broadway • (507) 292-7888 bluh2osalon.
com
Cloud 9 Spa & Salon F-5
112 1st Avenue SW • (507) 288-6689
massagecloud9.com

Healing Touch Spa F-5
111 S Broadway • (507) 287-6162 healingtouch-
rochester.com
Kahler Barbershop G-4
101 1st Avenue SW • (507) 282-4647
Rejuvenate Spa/Mayo Clinic Healthy Living
Program West of G-1
565 1st Street SW • (507) 293-2933
healthyliving.mayoclinic.org
Total Image Hair Salon G-4
20 2nd Avenue SW • (507) 289-4920

## TRANSPORTATION

### BUS

Rochester Public Transit
4300 E River Road NE • (507) 328-7433
rochesterbus.com

### CAR RENTAL

Avis G-4
20 2nd Avenue SW • (507) 288-5222 avis.com
Budget G-4
20 2nd Avenue SW • (507) 424-3377 budget.
com

### SHUTTLE

Groome Transportation F-1
821 Civic Center Drive NW
groometransportation.com/rochester
Rochester Shuttle Service G-4
20 2nd Avenue SW • (507) 216-6354
rochestershuttleservice.com

### TAXI

Med City Taxi
420 1st Avenue NW • (507) 282-8294
medcitytaxi.com
RST Taxi
25 9-1/2th Street SE • (507) 316-0955
Smart Ride Ecotaxi Pedicab
115 N Broadway • (507) 398-8009
gocarefreeshuttle.com
Yellow Cab
3736 Enterprise Drive SW • (507) 282-2222
yellowcabmedcity.com

# Index

Note: Page numbers in *italics* indicate maps/map descriptions.

CPSIA information can be obtained
at www.ICGtesting.com
Printed in the USA
LVHW051417161120
671798LV00010B/739